MW01037746

"This book can be a valuable resource for any medical student in navigating the sometimes tortuous waters of training in ways that will promote greater sanity, healing, and compassion, both for oneself, and for one's patients, not just while in school, but across the lifespan of one's practice." —JON KABAT-ZINN, PHD, Professor of Medicine emeritus, UMass Medical School, and author of *Coming to Our Senses: Healing Ourselves and the World Through Mindfulness*

"Jeremy Spiegel sees medical school as a process of discovery, in which students have the opportunity not only to study the mysteries of the human body but also psychological stress. *The Mindful Medical Student* offers concrete tips and exercises for dealing with the most common emotional pitfalls. In the process, Dr. Spiegel has managed to do what the other med school guides don't: treat the whole student. Don't go to med school without it." —SARA SKLAROFF, former editor of *U.S. News & World Report's Best Colleges* and *Best Graduate Schools* guidebooks

"This book is a wonderful, practical guide for medical students to become mindful, caring healers. Dr. Spiegel tells students how to combine mind, body, and spirit from the beginning of their training — an invaluable message." —JUDITH ORLOFF, MD, psychiatrist and author of *Positive Energy*

"Jeremy Spiegel's book is an excellent manual for medical students. It should be required reading for the first day of school, with revisits on holidays when there's time to breathe. Dr. Spiegel's introduction of mindfulness into medicine is essential and gives medical students a means to remember that they do care, which after all is why they want to be doctors." —LEWIS MEHL-MADRONA, MD, PHD, MPHIL, Associate Professor of Family Medicine and Psychiatry, University of Saskatchewan College of Medicine, and author of *Coyote Medicine* and *Narrative Medicine*

"Jeremy Spiegel's new text shines a useful and practical light on a great truth—it's important to stay true to yourself and the values that brought you to medicine during the difficult socialization process that is medical school. Dr. Spiegel gives practical strategies to both preserve your own humanity and share it with others as you mature into physicianhood. Having been a student affairs dean for years, I've never seen anything like this book. It is well worth reading and taking its lessons to heart for anyone on the journey to becoming a doctor." —JOSEPH F. O'DONNELL, MD, Senior Advising Dean and Director of Community Programs, Dartmouth Medical School

"*The Mindful Medical Student* is one of the rare books that seemingly focuses on a small group but has an appeal and very useful information for a much larger audience. The reader will find wisdom and guidance for the pursuit of one's dreams—all written in a most enjoyable style." —BARRY M. PANTER, MD, PHD, co-founder and director of The American Institute of Medical Education and The Creativity & Madness Conferences

"A thoughtful exploration of the emotional challenges posed by medical training, viewed from a psychoanalytic vantage. With dry wit, Dr. Spiegel offers a theoretical context for medical students' struggles and practical exercises to make the journey easier and more rewarding." —EMILY TRANSUE, MD, FACP, Clinical Assistant Professor of Medicine, University of Washington, and author of *On Call: A Doctor's Days and Nights in Residency* and *Patient by Patient*

The *Mindful*
Medical
Student

July 2015
To Ana Maria,
Thank you so much!
It was a pleasure
to meet you.
My best,
Jeremy Spiegel

JEREMY
SPIEGEL,
MD

foreword by
BERNIE SIEGEL,
MD

The *Mindful* Medical Student

A Psychiatrist's
Guide to Staying
Who You Are
While Becoming
Who You Want
to Be

dartmouth college press

hanover, new hampshire

published by

university press of new england

hanover and london

DARTMOUTH COLLEGE PRESS
Published by University Press of
New England, One Court Street,
Lebanon, NH 03766
www.upne.com
© 2009 by Jeremy Spiegel
Printed in U.S.A.
Designed and typeset in
Quadraat and Fresco Sans
by Eric M. Brooks

5 4 3 2 1

Library of Congress
Cataloging-in-Publication Data
Spiegel, Jeremy.
The mindful medical student: a
psychiatrist's guide to staying who
you are while becoming who you
want to be / Jeremy Spiegel.
    p.; cm.
Includes bibliographical references.
ISBN 978-1-58465-763-7
(pbk.: alk. paper)
1: Medical students — Life skill
guides. 2.Medical education —
Psychological aspects. I. Title.
[DNLM: I. Students, Medical —
psychology. 2. Education, Medical.
W 18 S755m 2009]
R737.S65   2009
610.71'1 — dc22   2008055185

University Press of New England
is a member of the Green Press
Initiative. The paper used in
this book meets their minimum
requirement for recycled paper.

Acknowledgments:
Adaptations of chapter 10,
"Dream Interpretation for First-
Time Scalpel Wielders," previously
appeared in Hot Psychology (July
2007) and The New Physician
(November 2007) magazines.

contents

foreword

The word *doctor* derives from the Latin word *docere*, which means "teacher." And it did not take me long to realize that we doctors really are here to teach—to educate people in how to live—and not just make diagnoses and write prescriptions.

Early in my career as a pediatric surgeon, a cancer patient taught me the importance of asking "How may I help you?" rather than "What's wrong with you?" Soon after, I found that doctors must learn to deal with loss rather than develop posttraumatic stress disorder due to all the pain we bury and never discuss on rounds or in conferences. These and other discoveries about the practice of medicine inspired in me a desire to help change medical schools from places that dispense information about disease and its treatment to places offering an education in caring for people.

In the hope of initiating such change, I wrote two letters, thirty years apart, to the respective deans of the medical school I attended, excerpts of which appear below:

April 7, 2007

Dear Dean Gotto,

I am writing to commend you on what you are doing to humanize medical care and education and help the students deal with their feelings too.

I cannot get the American College of Surgeons to change their pledge from "I will deal with my patients as I would wish to be dealt with" to "I will care for my patients as I would wish to be cared for."

My career was changed by [a] patient's request to help her to live between office visits. [In response,] I was criticized openly by many physicians and oncologists . . . about [my advocacy for] mind-body relationships, and so I was thrilled to see [it stated] in the alumni news, "We really are what we think."

One technique I use [to help humanize medical care] is to ask med students to draw themselves working as a doctor. Some drawings have no human beings in them, just instruments, books, and computers. Most reveal [a desk] and diplomas, with a doctor behind the desk. A rare picture shows true doctoring, handing a patient a tissue, and touching them with [a] hand and not a stethoscope. And I have yet to meet a med student who has been told, while in school, that Carl Jung, interpret[ing] a dream, . . . made a correct physical diagnosis.

I [also] believe enlightening the students about their true reasons for becoming physicians and analyzing them can help them . . . live a happier life when [people with] incurable [illnesses] show up as their patients. Most physicians suffer from PTSD and know how to think but not feel. Many famous paintings show doctors, chin in hand, thinking about a dying patient but never touching the patient.

So again, thank you, and if I can ever be of help in the humanizing process, please call upon me.

> Peace,
> Bernie Siegel, MD

March 1, 1977

Dear Dr. Meikle,

As I progress in the practice of medicine, I realize that the aspect I was least trained for is how to care for people and to establish a relationship with patients. We see more and more literature telling us how poorly we function, and indeed, I must agree with much of it. I am writing this letter in the hopes of having my thoughts be meaningful in the future development of physicians. . . .

I would hope that somewhere in the curriculum for the future, sociologists, humanitarians, and psychiatrists, as well as practicing physicians, can be involved in the development of the student's personality and . . . future dealings with human beings. I thought that in many areas my training was quite deficient and never really gave me a chance, aside from the obvious direct contact on wards, with the various problems and needs of the patients themselves. I have found that after being in practice I spent more time reading about patient-oriented problems than about the technical aspects of my trade. Yet, it is far easier to develop technical proficiency than proficiency in interpersonal relationships.

Having had the experience of being a patient shortly after entering practice, I would suggest, for whatever it is worth, having all future physicians spend a week in the hospital, perhaps with an IV taped to their arm, and limited to the assistance of those who will appear upon pushing the call button. I would feel that a week in this position would help to give them some realization of the complicated and stressful position that patients are in and the multiple needs that they have.

I hope that this letter [makes] some sense to you and frankly does not just represent an outpouring of my feelings, but a real desire to see us move forward in the area of physician training and teaching. I am very distressed with the situation I see around me, as . . . exists in some of our best hospitals, and find it difficult to sleep without making some effort to improve the situation.

Sincerely,

Bernard S. Siegel, MD

Neither dean wrote back. Had they replied, they would probably have agreed that students fascinated by the human body invariably have to deal with the fact that inside it there's a person.

That is why medical education must ultimately prepare students for the experience of caring for patients and not just dealing with their diseases.

If you are a medical student interested in becoming a caring doctor, you can begin through self-preparation. For starters, keep an open mind when exposing yourself to new subjects, such as end-of-life issues and integrative care, which organized medicine is only now beginning to explore. I hear doctors say "I can't accept that" when a new idea is incorporated into medical care. Similarly, when a student, focused on the interpersonal aspects of medicine, recently started a network called GEMS (Groups of Exceptional Medical Students), no one came to the initial meeting because they linked "exceptional" more to grades than to the willingness to relate to patients and their feelings.

In addition to keeping an open mind, analyze why you want to become a doctor. Acknowledge both the healthy and unhealthy reasons, so they will not interfere in patient care. If you tend toward perfectionism, remind yourself that we live in an imperfect world, which enriches our lives with meaning. If you experience pain in your interactions with patients, realize it is an outgrowth of your caring. A caring doctor means something in our world, because empathy and compassion are choices.

Finally, to prepare yourself for becoming an unceasingly caring doctor, read this book carefully. It can truly help you get ready for the *experience* of practicing medicine and also inspire you to create a mutual investment society with your patients. While living in your heart and not just your head, you can learn from your mortality how to engage fully in the time of your life.

BERNIE SIEGEL, MD

"Surgery is easy. It's relationships that are hard," a friend at my tenth medical school reunion confided to me, knowing that as a psychiatrist I had medical training and was accustomed to dealing with human behavior. I agreed that human interaction could be more difficult than the most complex medical procedures — say, neurosurgery. This exchange inspired me to consider the many emotional, psychological, and spiritual challenges medical school students face in addition to the usual course curricula and training. What were the common inner struggles, I wondered, that characterized a medical student's metamorphosis from pre–gross lab caterpillar to physician monarch butterfly?

Despite aptitude and enthusiasm for medical studies, I realized, at some time in the four years of medical school nearly every student gets caught in a web of confusion or anxiety about situations, patients, ideas, or personal reactions to ethical dilemmas. Such circumstances may cause uncertainty about behavior, raise questions about ethical conduct, provoke anxiety about proper role-playing, or even generate doubts about the suitability of a career in medicine.

Reflecting on my own experiences in medical school, I recalled that the emotional, psychological, and spiritual demands of my life as a medical student had indeed sometimes been harder than the intellectual challenges. While most new material about anatomy, differential diagnosis, or treatments had been reviewed so often it could be readily mastered, emotional struggles with medical issues, interpersonal relationships, and adaptation of personal traits to the medical school environment had often been problematic. Further, I had been ill-equipped for the inner conflicts produced by such situations and lacked the proper support or information necessary to maintain perspective.

As a result, in my third year of medical school I had what I now call an existential breakdown. I became increasingly aware of how truly different clinical rotations were from my previous academic work. Making sure to wash my hands thoroughly after cadaver class or letting my eyes relax enough to achieve stereoscopic vision through the binocular microscope in first- and second-year pathology lab were certainly minor achievements compared with what was expected of me in my clerkships. During one of my first rotations, I experienced a condition of disabling demoralization that reached crisis status. The hospital's din of retching and bells, and the general disarray, emotional intensity, and huge number of patients all in such a confined area were dizzying and almost unbearable. With stress and pain all around me, as well as within me, I felt lost in the desolate moonscape of the internal medicine ward. I struggled to maintain my sense of identity and ethics amid challenging interactions with staff and patients, and attempted in vain to blame others for my unfortunate predicament. Moreover, I was skeptical about training to become like some of the medical personnel who were supposedly my role models and concerned that my personality was changing in a way that did not bode well for a promising future. Consequently, I had trouble fathoming how satisfying it would eventually be to work as a physician.

After deferring my medicine rotation for four weeks to do some soul searching, I gradually began to comprehend that I could learn how to resolve emotional, psychological, and spiritual dilemmas through trial and error, inner reflection, and using other medical personnel advantageously—if not as role models then as guides to assist in determining my own views and direction. As I began acting on the insights I had gained, it became increasingly clear that medical school does not create doctors;

rather, medical students must transform themselves into doctors by using their own inner resources in addition to the information and expertise they absorb from their training.

Reflecting on this time of trial, I realize that it would have helped to have had access to the critical "emotional education" I needed to complement the required intellectual learning. Then I would have had more warning and guidance about the kinds of emotional and psychological challenges I could expect as a medical student. Further, I recognize the role that psychiatry can play in helping not just patients but also fellow physicians and future physicians as they face the many challenges of the medical profession.

My aim in this book is to offer valuable insights for the current generation of medical students. Since in my medical school career I learned more from the broad thinkers than from the "walking encyclopedias," it focuses on self-discovery and facing the emotional, psychological, and spiritual challenges of medical school rather than on facts. Any medical student can use Google to find bits of data when the computer behind the nurse's station is finally free, but it is more difficult to obtain concrete guidance for inner struggles. Because I learned most from doctors willing to be real about the experience of medicine rather than only singing its praises, this book also gives honest appraisals of potential problems and offers possible solutions to assist medical students in seeing the reality of medical school instead of some idealized vision. Another practical aspect of the book is its numerous stories and hands-on exercises that increase awareness of potential solutions to critical emotional, psychological, ethical, and spiritual dilemmas arising in medical settings. I hope that this book will provide helpful personal guideposts for students seeking to find their way in medical school and beyond.

introduction

What is the sound of one
latex-gloved hand clapping?

The Mindful Medical Student is a guide
to dealing with the emotional, psychological, ethical, and spiritual challenges of medical school and a career in medicine. It
complements the intellectual and technical curriculum of medical school by providing crucial information and advice about
issues of personal identity, interpersonal relationships, ethical
dilemmas, and other causes of inner conflicts. The goal is an enlightened self, an individual who is more capable of searching
within for answers, behaving more consciously, engaging with
others more knowingly, and emerging stronger from any tribula-
tion during medical school and beyond.

Although the term mindful is taken from Zen Buddhist practice, the use of Eastern tenets, such as meditation, is only one
aspect of being a mindful medical student. Such students also
have a broader humanistic outlook on life and are thus thoughtful, caring, and empathetic to the self, patients, and others. They
have explored the self sufficiently to know personal strengths and
weaknesses and to not let the chaotic and challenging circumstances of medical school threaten their identity or progress in
the medical profession. Instead, through increased awareness of
their circumstances and coping techniques, they ensure that they
become the compassionate, effective physicians they envision.

Because medical schools focus on conveying clinical knowledge and skills, there is insufficient acknowledgment that they

are also social arenas in which people with diverse personas, roles, and agendas can complicate training or that the pressures of medical school can exacerbate student psychological or emotional problems. Unlike solitary academic life in a carrel on C floor of the university library, medical school forces students to embrace teamwork—a requirement that requires each student to interact effectively with many different types of people, including difficult peers, authoritarian medical "elders," and stubborn patients, while, hopefully, refusing to take on their negative qualities. Also, much as patients with posttraumatic stress disorder feel alienated from their surroundings and themselves, and thus lose perspective or experience delusions or emotional trauma, medical students can face such problems as anxiety, obsessions, perfectionism, acting out, difficulty in relating to people, burnout, emotional shutdown, and depression.

The best defenses against allowing such problems to impede your progress toward a thriving career in medicine are increased awareness and effective tools. A recent study on the well-being of medical students, published in the journal *Academic Medicine*, concluded that "medical schools need to educate students about the variety of personal and professional stressors experienced during training and inform them how to access resources" and recommended that medical schools provide students with skills needed to assess personal distress, determine its effect on their care of patients, recognize when they need assistance, and develop strategies to promote their own well-being (Dyrbye et al., 2006, 380). Like the psychiatrist has his interview, the surgeon her scalpel and Debakey clamp, the allergist his scratch test, and the gastroenterologist her endoscope, you as a medical student can learn to rely on your inner self to master people skills, broaden your perspective, and draw upon insights gleaned through reflection.

Thus the goal of the information and tools presented in this book is to promote self-awareness, self-regulation, and self-healing. Even if guidance from others in medical school, or from an outside therapist or psychiatrist, becomes necessary, your investment in self-education will increase your ability to care for yourself at the most trying times in your training.

Despite its focus on the self, the program outlined in this book is not intended as an isolated venture, and in fact addresses ways to nurture relationships with peers as an invaluable resource. It also advocates learning from the experiences of former medical students, examples of which are included, as well as from the thoughts and actions of fictional characters in stories and plays. "Triangle of Medicine" diagrams, appearing in chapters 3 and 5, provide a handy mnemonic device for maintaining awareness of the complex interpersonal forces underlying every medical interaction. Much as you would work out in the gym, you can use the advice, stories, and exercises in this book to ground yourself, take care of yourself, and re-create yourself for the greatest possible success in medical school and beyond.

Discovering Who You Are

You begin your life as a medical student by focusing on intellectual tasks—having achieved excellence in academics by filling in the correct bubbles with number-two pencils. Although you are trained to synthesize new data and absorb centuries' worth of specialized knowledge about the workings of the human body, your book smarts are of limited value if you lack a good understanding of your broader emotional and psychological self and how your own and others' behavior can affect the progress of your medical training. Whether you're at the beginning of medical training or have already completed a few clinical rotations, you can improve your chances of success by transforming yourself from a walking, talking brain into the broader soma vital for good doctoring. Discovering who you are and learning how to remain connected to your true, or authentic, self throughout the challenging days of medical school can help you stay on track to become the effective and compassionate doctor you have envisioned yourself being. Part I of this book introduces significant features of your emotional and psychological self and provides tools for gaining a greater awareness of their importance for positive achievement in medical school and later in the medical profession.

Chapter 1, "Finding Your True Self," focuses on the skill of listening to yourself to identify the true nature of your character and explains why remaining connected to your true self is advantageous in medical school. Further, this chapter shows how to educate your inner self in tandem with your external medical education to nurture your true self. It also includes suggestions for adhering to your true self during times of stress or when facing ethical dilemmas or problematic interpersonal relationships.

Chapter 2, "Gaining Awareness of Your False Self," explores the origins and agendas of your false self and reveals how easily thoughts and attitudes derived from your false self, instead of your true self, can negatively affect your work in medical school. Tips are given on how to identify aspects of your false self, how to avoid letting them influence your behavior, how to remain consistent—and thus in tune with your true self—and how to develop your capacity to feel compassion toward others and yourself by attending to your own needs. This chapter provides techniques for evaluating distortions of the true self and visual meditation for maintaining positive attitudes conducive to repudiating your false self.

Chapter 3, "Tuning In to Acting Out," illustrates how your behavior may compromise your future in medicine when you lose sight of your true self and allow stressful situations to irritate old wounds or make you reenact old conflicts. Further, it illustrates how, without your fingers on the pulse of your true self, you can activate defense mechanisms that are disadvantageous for learning and ultimately impede your progress in medical school.

Methods are provided for recognizing how you may be acting out and ways to avoid such behavior.

Chapter 4, "Grappling with Perfectionism and Obsessive-Compulsive Behavior," addresses some of the potentially debilitating habits that may have been useful for the MCAT but could prevent your effective participation as a full-fledged member of a medical team. Techniques are offered for recognizing and treating yourself should problematic behavior emerge.

1 Finding Your True Self

An important key to success in medical school can be summed up in the directive "Adhere closely to your true, or authentic, self and it will lead you in the right direction." Adhering to your true self means being real, permitting yourself to experience genuine feelings, and acting according to your fundamental character and principles. However, because medical school challenges individuality and causes stress through routines, rigorous training, and control by superiors, it can easily disconnect you from your true self and thus from its inherent wisdom — wisdom that is a great asset in such a setting.

Determination to discover and nurture your true self from day one of medical school will help you access feelings directly, remain untainted by others' views or agendas, and be an open-minded thinker and humane healer. When connected to your true self, you are guided not from without — by parents, fellow students, residents, and attending physicians — but from within, from aspects of yourself that reflect your natural inclinations, deepest beliefs and feelings, and sense of purpose. And when, in addition, you are nourished emotionally, psychologically, or spiritually by beneficial relationships, stimulating interests, or transcendent experiences, your true self grows stronger and thus becomes an even more reliable foundation for rewarding accomplishments in medicine.

Your true self is found by peeling away layers of traits and behaviors that have resulted from the influence of others, like coats of paint scraped away to reveal the brilliant, life-sized gold heart that is your essence. This heart contains personal truths that will be revealed to you only as you actively search for your personal interests, ideals, hopes, and dreams, all of which may have been obscured over the years leading up to medical school by such factors as parents' demands and expectations, societal pressures, and peer influences.

One method of discovering more about your true self is to ask yourself the following three questions on a daily basis. Doing so helps you become increasingly better able to distinguish between when you are deviating from your natural inclinations and sense of purpose and when you are following the dictates of your true self while interacting with a patient, the patient's family, residents, attendings, or people you care about at home.

1 *Do I recognize myself?* Despite the frenetic pace of your new life, in quiet moments literally look for reflections of yourself as a way to access and reinforce your true self. For example, while in the hospital cafeteria you may be able to glimpse your reflection on the back of a spoon or in the taut Saran Wrap before it is removed from the cup of pudding; or on the ward at night you may perhaps see your face in the turned-off TV screen or in the window while helping a patient. This simple technique of face-image association offers opportunities for discovering your true self through asking further questions, such as *Do I recognize this person as my true self? Is what I am doing (thinking, saying) today consistent with who I have always been?* If you feel you are embracing a new self-image, then you can ask yourself additional questions to determine its origins and whether you like or dislike it. Such questions will often initiate an important dialogue with your true self that can help refine your understanding of it.

For example, often, as he walked between the intensive care unit and the step-down unit, Taylor was riddled with doubts about himself, especially his physical ability to perform procedures on live human patients. From time to time, he used the shiny, white corridor with its reflective walls as a mirror to discover aspects of his true self. Soon he noticed a transformation of himself that became disconcerting. He explained, "The old me—usually very flexible, curious, and capable—became blended with this new person I saw in the reflection, this older, tired-looking figure wearing my coat and hospital badge, which felt like a kind of costume. I found myself getting short and snappy, and I knew there was a perpetual expression on my face that read 'stress.' Sitting in the conference hall awaiting the start of didactics, I thought about what I saw in myself. I knew that I was now different. I realized that it was the stress of being near younger burn patients that was having an effect on me. After that I continued looking at myself daily as a way to return to the usual me."

2 *Whose voice am I using?* When you speak to others, take note of whether your attitude, words, and tone are consistent with the kind of person you have always been. If you notice a new trait, ask yourself who influenced it and whether you like it. Observing yourself this way can make you conscious of external influences that might be affecting you, even if subconsciously.

For instance, when a chief resident in general surgery I once worked with bemoaned the universal need for lunch as annoying to "progress," a medical student sitting across the table from him agreed with this absurd argument. Later, the student was able to identify the influence on his view when he caught himself parroting the resident's attitudes of workaholism and self-importance—views that previously had been foreign to him. He had been so caught up in the thrill of his new rotation that he had let himself be molded by an authority figure, even playing a role when he came home in the evening to his wife. In instances when it is not possible or appropriate to contradict a medical "elder's" view in public, you can make a mental note to later reaffirm your own beliefs with yourself, family, and friends.

3 *Am I disavowing something important to me?* When a supervisor's recommendation jars your sensibilities, this most likely signals that the suggested action might be at odds with your true self. Such a signal is like an indicator light on your psychic dashboard that grows in luminescence the more your self-awareness increases. Consequently, when you get such a signal, use it to discover more about your true self by evaluating its potential implications in light of how you have defined your true self.

Another good way to discover your true self is by intentionally spending time alone. Solitude for self-discovery may work best in a nature setting, but if there is no park nearby and the only options are a shopping mall, the inside of your car, or a supermarket, choose the one offering the fewest distractions. Then, among the trees or the stacks of soup cans, remind yourself that you are an organism guided by instincts, visual cues, and intuition. Notice what encourages you to take one path over another — such as types or shapes of objects and their links to specific feelings. Recognize what inspires good feelings and its potential sources in childhood experiences. Realize aspects about you that have endured despite the passage of time and provided a foundation for qualities developed later. By repeatedly going on these types of quasi–spirit quests you will gradually unearth the basic characteristics and beliefs of your true self.

Yet another method for discovering your true self is to go to an art museum and pick out one work of art that most closely resembles your inner life. In looking for it, you essentially will be searching for your true self, becoming, in the process, more conscious of your likes and dislikes, strengths and weaknesses, and hopes and dreams. Is it a Mondrian with rectangles and few colors, a Picasso or Braque cubist piece, a politically charged Jenny Holzer, a photograph, or a pre-Columbian figure seeming to stare into space? Once you have selected the work of art that most reflects your true self, sit in front of it and meditate on it or sketch it on a small card. You might even imagine the serpent of the caduceus wending its way through your work, taking note of all the relevant colors, forms, and figures along its path. In this way you can learn how to incorporate into yourself its symbols, making your own insignias that can be useful later for reference. Then you can conjure it up in the form of a mental image or, if you have sketched it, keep the card in your pocket to look at from time to time for inspiration, comfort, and a standard by which to determine whether or not you are adhering to your true self in your present endeavors.

A final way to discover your true self is to imagine your own face in place of a dying patient's face or your medical school cadaver's face, and then consider what you would like to accomplish before your death. In particular, determine the aspects of life most significant to you, the traits you regard as fundamental to your character, and the dreams you have had that stand out as essential for future fulfillment.

After discovering your true self, consider how various factors specific to medical training can inhibit its expression. In this chapter, we will briefly explore six such factors. One is postponement of gratification, which is considered a requirement for academic achievement. Pre-med students, particularly science majors, become accustomed to waiting for an uncertain payoff, especially while painstakingly running experiments and analyzing results. They have all waited for something to grow in a beaker or for a centrifuge to slow down before removing the tubes; patiently titrated solutions in the chemistry lab; waited for bacteria to incubate, DNA strands to replicate, or proteins to migrate across a polarized gel. Clever management of time and a high threshold for frustration accompany such pursuits. In fact, the entire protracted course of medical training entails persistence, or what psychiatrists lightheartedly refer to as "stick-to-it-iveness." However, this capacity to delay gratification, while advantageous for short-term success as a student and likely to pay off professionally, comes at a considerable cost to the expression of your true self.

Therefore, as a medical student it is especially important to balance delayed gratification with nurturing of the true self. For example, any time it is inappropriate to act on your needs and desires, you could quietly observe them, honoring them by maintaining awareness of them or even talking to yourself about them. *I'm hungry*, you might say to yourself after spending an hour and a half with your neck craned over the eyepieces of a microscope. *I'm discouraged*, you might admit after a study session with a phone book–sized encyclopedia of cells and tissues. *I'm bored, and I miss my girlfriend (boyfriend, friend, mother)*, you tell yourself while hunched over a sterile carrel in the micropathology section of the library, well past any reasonable person's bedtime. Commenting to yourself about your needs helps you not only maintain awareness of them but also forge an alliance with your true self and thus stand your ground against masochistic study-marathons and demoralizing self-denying behaviors.

Another factor that can impede expression of the true self is differences in opinion or attitude between you and those charged with teaching you. Authority figures such as teachers, administrators, and attending physicians frequently pressure medical students to adopt the prevailing views to facilitate teamwork or to justify their own authoritative status. For example, at one medical school's orientation week a nationally recognized physician turned the classical version of the Hippocratic oath into a personal polemic when, during his keynote address to the incoming class, he used it to lend authority to his own bias against euthanasia and abortion—a sobering signal to his students of the need to stay connected to their true selves throughout the four years ahead. No matter what your view or how contentious the topic, at medical school you will encounter potential conflict between the opinions of authority figures projected in loud voices and your own views existing quietly in the mind of "just a face in the lecture hall." To avoid feeling intimidated by authority figures and losing your sense of being a creative individual and an independent thinker, it is essential to connect with your true self periodically, reassuring yourself that you do not need to give up your own views and desires merely because someone with greater experience is expressing different ones. To reinforce this sense of individuality, it may help to split your world mentally into two columns: "me" versus "not me," practicing awareness of the distinction between the two to nourish your true self.

A third factor that can inhibit expression of the true self in medical school is sheer lack of time. With constant requirements and obligations, it is difficult to devote time to activities that nourish the true self, like reading for pleasure, playing sports, working at hobbies you are passionate about. To overcome this drawback, you could learn to acknowledge your needs and desires during stressful times and devise ways to incorporate personal activities into your routine by reducing the time allotted to them or keeping objects related to them in view. For instance, you might manage to squeeze knitting or pick-up basketball into your schedule or, as a reminder of your passion for sports or painting, keep the equipment required for them visible to nurture your true self. Ironically, unstructured time allows you to be more effective and productive, the same way a mini-vacation refreshes you so you can continue to work without burning out.

Stress is yet another factor that often inhibits expression of the true self in medical school, since a relaxed frame of mind is usually required to access the true self. To deal with this problem, you can practice stress-reducing exercises (various forms of meditation or other relaxation techniques) and learn to condense such techniques so they can be better interspersed with your hectic daily activities. For example, while practicing relaxation at home, undisturbed, you can link your relaxed state with a "trigger" phrase that can be used later to induce that state during stressful times in medical situations. One approach is that while sitting comfortably in a quiet place, focused on breathing effortlessly from your abdomen, a hand on your chest and another your abdomen, you can link a two-word phrase to your relaxed state by thinking something like *Let go* or *I'm floating*. Then later, in the frenzy of the ward or before an exam, instead of disappearing into the equipment room every time you get tense, you can repeat silently to yourself the two-word phrase practiced at home and thus conjure up those same feelings of relaxation. With practice, you'll be able to relax using your trigger phrase as if you had antistress medication in your pocket, but without side effects, drug-drug interactions, or limitations on refills.

An additional factor that can inhibit expression of the true self is second-guessing yourself, a habit that can become magnified in medical school because of the great expectations medical students must try to fulfill. Without confidence in your own observations, reasoning, and choices, you likely will succumb to the tide of information and opinions washing over you from your medical training. A knee-jerk deferral toward others with more education, experience, and authority undermines and devalues your true self. For example, Eli struggled with staying open-minded enough to permit a wide-ranging list of possible conditions while developing a differential diagnosis for a case with his team. Because he had difficulty permitting himself to be wrong, he tended to ignore the important practice of making diagnoses by first using a wide net and then gradually ruling out possibilities, and instead was quick to espouse a single diagnosis to avoid the too-familiar pain of second-guessing himself. By holding on tightly to one possibility with his mind shut, Eli opted for narrow thinking and effectively dissociated from his true self. As a result, curiosity, exploration, and creative outside-the-box thinking were all discarded when he, like many medical students, cut himself off from the process of learning and, as a consequence, of good doctoring.

Finally, a major stumbling block to expressing your true self in medical school is burnout, particularly caregiver burnout. This can occur especially when you have to take care of one of your own family members on top of your duties caretaking in medical settings; for instance, when your spouse or parent is emotionally needy, seeks medical advice, or requires in-home care—or some energy-sapping combination of these. You—as a busy medical student requiring intense focus and freedom from outside pressures—like the old song, "do not have time for the pain," and yet your typical medical student "natural helper" personality predisposes you to try to fix or manage all situations simultaneously, resulting in a loss of your true self.

Such a dilemma occurred to one of the most generous people in her medical class, Katie, whose mother had been diagnosed with lupus, a perplexing disorder of the immune system. Seeing her daughter as a doctor already, Katie's mother called her three times a week, with many often-unanswerable medical questions, and also desperately sought emotional support. Although initially intrigued with the notion that she might be able to impart valuable medical knowledge and help her mother, Katie's efforts were eventually transformed into masochistic drudgery that threatened her wish for a career. She began to question her tolerance for dealing with patients' afflictions and felt that features of her true self, such as her zest for medicine and natural curiosity, were becoming undermined by caregiving burnout.

After you have used any of these methods to access and define your true self and have a greater awareness of how medical school experiences can inhibit its expression, it is important to learn more about how to nurture it and regularly maintain your connection to it during challenging times in medical school. These are skills that can be learned, then practiced. Like a seasoned yogi who can regulate his heart rate using only the power of his mind, you can access and nurture your true self to sustain and guide you during times of crisis in the lecture hall, the seminar room, or on the ward, whether you are in the throes of your class's collective pretest anxiety, facing your resident's acerbic criticism, or engaged in a spiritually demanding encounter with a dying patient. By committing to a few moments daily with your true self, such as meditating on the subway, listing your desires in a notebook on your night table, or visualizing your dreams while on the elliptical machine—you will be more self-assured in facing the constant challenges of medical school.

One good way to nurture and maintain your true self is by keeping a journal or by writing creatively to express your inner thoughts and feelings, about both your past and present, to gain perspective. Think, for example, of a major conflict in your past and write about its significance in light of your fundamental character and life goals. Next, consider whether any conflicts in medical school are related to it. Finally, write about ways you can deal with the current conflict and still maintain your fundamental character and life goals. Such personal history mining and examination allow you more easily to keep yourself fixed within the realm of your true self, since any present conflicts are not experienced in a vacuum but can be recognized as familiar patterns from the past. Thus your mind will register them not as threatening, live viruses but instead as spirit- and stamina-strengthening inoculations. This concept represents the core paradigm of psychodynamic psychotherapy: situations in a person's current life that cause emotional distress relate to something particularly evocative from the past. Old conflicts, feelings, and situations find new life in present stress, particularly when the stress is as great as it is in medical school.

You can also nurture and maintain your true self by expressing your feelings to others. One medical student reported having the following pivotal experience during an internal medicine rotation:

> I admitted a young man in his early twenties, who, per the history gathered from the patient's family and from the police report, was pulled over on the highway for presumed DWI. He had been weaving on the road, was stopped, and given the usual sobriety tests. The officers thought something was wrong with their Breathalyzer when he blew a .000. Later they confirmed with toxicology screens that there was not a trace of alcohol or illicit drugs in the patient's system.
>
> When I admitted him, we scanned his head and the CT revealed something horrible. There in front of us all was this monster—a lesion in his brain like I had never seen before. This inoperable tumor in a person not much younger than myself was more disturbing than anything I had dealt with before in my life. And somehow either I was persuaded or I volunteered to break this tragic news to the family. I will never forget their faces while straining to see through my teary eyes.
>
> I later told the attending and the medicine chief resident that I didn't know if I really had what it took to deal with one tragedy after another, and was growing uncertain about my career choice. But one immediately said, "No, you're a natural, there's no question of that." Hearing this reaffirmed my sense of identity as an aspiring doctor.

These empathetic momentary mentors recognized the positive qualities of the medical student, most likely because the student let himself be real, feeling the horror of the family's grief and later expressing his true emotions with his attending and resident. As a result, they could see that he was an individual in the process of becoming a high-caliber doctor and, through their words of encouragement, could reinforce the qualities of his true self.

Thus, ironically, maintaining your true self and letting yourself emerge as a natural healer might be done more easily in the context of tragedy, such as while identifying with a terminal patient or his grieving family members, as Gregory David Roberts, a self-trained physician in the slums of Bombay, India, observed in his book *Shantaram*: "It's a characteristic of human nature that the best qualities, called up quickly in a crisis, are very often the hardest to find in a prosperous calm. The contours of all our virtues are shaped by adversity" (379). Just as the author came to know and nurture his true self while treating cholera, dodging feline-sized rats, and suturing gaping lacerations, you can nurture your true self by maintaining awareness of your feelings and sensations in times of medical challenges and crises.

This is exemplified by the honest way Roberts describes suturing skin: "Human skin is tougher and more resilient than it looks. It's also relatively simple to stitch, and the thread can be pulled quite tightly without tearing the tissue. But the needle, no matter how fine or sharp, is still a foreign object, and for those of us who aren't inured to such work through frequent repetition, there's a psychological penalty that must be paid each time we drive that alien thing into another being's flesh" (307). Roberts emerges as physician not because of what he stitches, but because of his empathy and an internal calling to heal, qualities that derive from maintaining a connection to the true self.

Finding your true self and then nourishing it so it will always be accessible is a profound way to begin advocating for yourself and refining your talents as a healer. Soon you will be able to braid together your book knowledge, clinical experience, and the wisdom of your true self in a kind of lanyard that can be worn around your neck like an amulet, providing strength and protection in the stressful situations that occur throughout the years of medical school.

2 | Gaining Awareness of Your False Self

Despite your best efforts to maintain loyalty to your true self, in medical school you may at times confront a false self in various guises. The false self arises from interactions with the outside world, while the true self originates from within. The false self is like a gram-negative rod that either colonizes or dies, depending on the relative nutritive value of its growing medium. In the thick agar of your new stressful microenvironments—lectures, labs, and rotations—ugly aspects of your false self can emerge, gain strength, and overshadow your true self's desires. In this way, your false self can derail you from your otherwise well-intentioned, high-minded goal of becoming a valued and successful physician.

An emerging false self that is difficult to detect can lead to potentially dangerous problems. Something as simple as a bad attitude can develop into jaded cynicism or outright rebellion. For instance, activation of the false self can make a student inclined to organize a quiet coup in the pathology lab, while another might "get off" on being a scrubs-shrouded hotshot, who, using her motley assemblage of patients as a kind of foil, disgracefully bolsters her self-image at the expense of compassionate action. A physician named Patrick remembers when the small group of his first-year medical school peers, selfishly looking out for their own interests, hid slides of fatty liver and the caseating granuloma of tuberculosis prior to a micropathology examination so the other students wouldn't be able to identify the associated diseases. The culprits' actions, while not impeding the success of the other students, reflected an underlying bad attitude that seemed inconsistent with the qualities of their true selves and of physicians in training.

Circumstances on the ward may actually foster the emergence of one's false self. Tom, a clever and self-assured third-year medical student, seemed to be really enthusiastic about his rotations except that he parroted, with a kind of disdain, what he heard cynical residents saying, calling patients "gomers" (get out of my emergency room), or using such expressions as (the classic reductio ad insultum) "the liver" or "the kidney" or "the heart in Room 102." Although the use of such jargon might make it appear that Tom was only trying to integrate himself into the medical scene, his parroting of pseudosophisticated, cynical phrases was masking his true self as he assumed a role. These are examples of the false self encouraging a bad attitude; and such attitudes can lead to real problems, like acting on negative thoughts — for instance, holding unexpurgated impromptu roasts with your residents outside patients' hospital rooms. By observing the behaviors of others and assessing your own behavior, you can more readily identify the difference between your true and false selves, understand the destructive potential of your false self, learn to avoid its pitfalls, and maintain a healthy connection to your true self.

A good way, then, to avoid giving in to behavior reflecting your false self is to objectively assess whether or not your thoughts and actions are aligned with who you have been, who you are, and who you want to be. When the shotgun spray of points on your scatter plot denotes a hornet's nest of negativity, or you express extreme optimism in the face of calamity, you likely are being internally inconsistent, unaligned with your true self.

Another indication of the false self is insensitivity to patients. For example, morbid fascination with a person's presenting illness — a grapefruit-sized tumor, beach ball–sized abdominal ascites, or hideous teratoma — likely reflects emerging aspects of your false self. While interest in exploring medical pathology may serve you and your patients well at times, fascination that gravitates toward excitement when someone's organs are splayed out before you, and the patient's fate hangs on your every word and action, reflects your false self. In such instances you are being internally inconsistent and relatively unaware of the dissonance between your intellectual stimulation and the feelings of your not-so-enthusiastic patient. The more inclined you are to treat your patient as a specimen, the more you become like a Frankenstein, who, while giving life to several pounds of recovered flesh, lost his own humanity in the process.

One way to detect the emergence of your false self is by assessing whether your thoughts and actions are consistent with your true self as you know it. When you start behaving in ways you consider "not you" more often than acting in a manner you consider "you," this is a sign that your false self is becoming dominant. One medical student, Nancy, became increasingly aware of her thoughts changing. Due to the stress of her position on the lowest rung of the medical totem pole, she found herself frequently putting people down in her mind. She soon began to realize that her attitude shift was unhelpful in situations where people's lives were on the line.

One medical student, Sam, gained awareness of how the false self can lead to insensitivity to patients. In a twist of fate, his wife's grandmother became a patient during his medicine rotation. Sam, recalling his initially conflicting feelings about the situation, said:

What's weird is that I didn't speak up about knowing this person in Room 112A, a grandmotherly figure who lives — literally, as in the fairy tale — in the woods among her chickens and outbuildings, including a little house dedicated to quilting activities. Why I wasn't moved to mention my connection to her I don't know, but this did something to my perspective. All of a sudden, the kind of artifice created here, the "us" versus "them," the doctors versus the patients, that had appealed to me at first didn't feel right to me after Grammy hit the ward. When they called out her last name, it really did something that eluded my full understanding. This was not Mrs. So-and-So, I wanted to say, this was Grammy and I'm worried about her.

I was worried also that even some of the more gentle mocking—the harmless rhyming and limerick-making using patients' strange-sounding names, or the rude commentary on patients' unflattering physical features or idiosyncrasies—might occur outside her room. So I felt tense and in a protective mode, ready to hush anyone who dared to make me feel badly about someone I cared about. As it turns out, my fears were not realized, and when I gave her a kiss and they could see plainly that I knew her, I felt like I had thrown an invisible cloak of protection around her. Fortunately, she left the hospital not long after her diagnosis of viral meningitis and recovered well.

After this incident, Sam made more of an effort to remain in touch with his true self when around patients. Although he continued to use humor to soothe his own and others' stress and occasionally flipped a rhyme, this encounter served as a kind of inoculation against false-self venom. He swore to remember that every person he treated was someone else's grandmother, father, daughter, son, mother, or lover, and that that person deserved the best from those entrusted to care for him or her.

After observing situations in which aspects of your false self are at play and learning to identify those aspects, for greater understanding of how to minimize their power, it is important to search for their origins. Features of the false self can invariably be traced back to old personal shortcomings and emotional wounds that have surfaced due to stress or the recurrence of previously traumatic circumstances. As an illustration: One physician remembers an intense reaction he had to a patient who weighed three hundred pounds, glistened with sweat, exuded a sickly odor, and produced an impressive sample of intertriginous cheese, discovered during daily physical examinations. The doctor, while aware that he was supposed to be professional, couldn't help being repulsed by the man. Although by itself this was not necessarily alarming—indeed, it can be a stress reliever to think negative thoughts about a patient that you would not dare utter aloud—the doctor's repulsion had become so habitual it was affecting his medical assessments of the patient's condition. At last the doctor managed to connect his repulsion to a childhood fear of a fat person, at which point his feelings stopped affecting his judgments.

Explaining the origins of the false self even more specifically, psychiatrists D. W. Winnicott and R. D. Laing state that the false self likely originates from the concealing or betraying of one's own true possibilities. Because the false self arises from relationship with the outside world, it often becomes a conduit for the expression of the person's psychological wounds. Laing, in his book *The Divided Self*, wrote, regarding a patient whose false self was empowered by suppressed needs and wishes, "All that could not find expression and open acknowledgment in her was condensed in her presenting symptoms" (110).

To deflate the ballooning power of your false self, then, it is necessary to look within yourself to uncover traumas, hurts, attitudes, and family myths that have been important in your life. In her classic work, *The Drama of the Gifted Child*, Alice Miller highlights the value of recognizing and feeling directly "the resentment and mourning aroused by our parents' failure to fulfill our primary needs" (20). Unless they are examined closely, these emotional injuries become fodder for the false self and are easily used against those who are most vulnerable—namely, coworkers and patients. This search may be complicated by the fact that academically successful, gifted, motivated individuals, such as those who make it into medical school, usually remain off the radar screen of guidance personnel and thus emotional wounds can go undetected, while a student whose grades drop might receive counseling more readily.

If they are not consciously explored, a medical student's emotional wounds might sporadically surface while he's negotiating the stress of medical school, as one medical student experienced. Howard's parents, both practicing physicians, created an environment for their son that made it difficult for him to express his true self. As a youth, he spent too many potential play-hours alone in his room fingering his violin—an instrument chosen for him by his misguided but well-meaning parents. In addition, his parents tended to discount his feelings. "You don't feel that way," Howard's mom would frequently respond to any point of view at odds with her perspective on things. To deal with his distaste for stringed instruments and other impositions, Howard developed a false self, which soon made him feel alienated or, as he described it, "not real, like on some kind of life-treadmill with the stop button missing." Later, his false self surfaced under stress in medical school; for instance, when it came time to give opinions on the ward, he became stunned, like a deer in oncoming headlights. Eventually, upon realizing the origins of this false self and the emotional toll of unquestioningly following others' well-intentioned guidance for him, he managed to cast off the constraints of his false self. Through reflection and use of the technique of face-image association (see chapter 1), he begin living life with more of a connection to his own feelings.

To free yourself from false-self shackles and avoid later acting out, it is necessary to identify and acknowledge existing emotional wounds and then declare your intention of self-healing. First, find a place where you might stare at yourself in a mirror or other reflective surface while sitting comfortably. As you stare at your face, relax to the point where you start to look a little differ-ent—in the same way the spelling of a word appears odd if you focus on it for too long. Now, while looking at yourself, gaze into the pain and unease that found refuge within you. To enhance your ability to visualize the resulting inner wounds, you might play some music that moves you, or surround yourself with in-spirational pictures of a scene or object that represents some struggle or pain from your past. Then ask yourself, *What do I see that I do not like? What are my emotional wounds?* Like the light from stars whose beams travel widely divergent spans of time to meet your retinas in a single glance, such a view of yourself unifies past with present. Next, let the players emerge who had a role in shaping the "you" that you now face. Give back to them any hurt-ful comments, inattention to your true feelings, falseness you de-veloped within yourself as a means of surviving the oppressive framework of their needs and desires. If you wish, vocalize this as an official pronouncement of its finality, using phrases such as, "Here, I give you back my _____ (insecurity, ugly com-petitiveness, desperation to be liked), for which I no longer have any use. Thank you."

As you practice this technique, you may discover more deeply embedded emotional wounds, as though peeling layers of an onion. For inspiration, you could consider artists who have fo-cused on self-revelation, such as Chuck Close, who spent de-cades revealing aspects of himself through brilliant self-portrai-ture. The more you discover, the more you can subdue aspects of your false self that undermine your positive development during medical school and beyond.

Interestingly, while the false self uses emotional wounds to undermine development and harmonious relationships with others, the true self utilizes emotional wounds to enhance devel-opment and harmonious relationships with others—provided the emotional wounds have been acknowledged and deeply felt instead of disavowed. An example of this dynamic appears in the

Thornton Wilder play *The Angel That Troubled the Waters*, brought to my attention by noted surgeon and author Bernie Siegel. In it, a physician learns that the anguish of his own personal pain becomes his greatest asset in the care of patients and their families. Like the physical wounds of scarification given to young people in tribal initiation rites, such emotional wounds can be healed, strengthening the deeper personality of the individual. For illustration, a doctor grappling with emotional wounds rooted in his experience of Tourette's syndrome—characterized by facial grimaces and vocal tics—discovered through his struggle a surprising interaction between himself and patients. Even slight tics seemed to have a positive effect on his patients, making it easier to identify with him as not just doctor but also patient, thus setting a tone for compassion and healing.

Doctors with unacknowledged emotional wounds, on the other hand, tend not to foster harmonious patient relationships. For instance, a doctor who disavows his emotional wounds related to an intractable eating disorder and who appears sick with swollen parotid glands and a sallow complexion does not instill empathy or confidence in healing.

In addition to uncovering emotional wounds, another way to disempower your false self during medical interactions is to have a compassionate stance toward yourself. No one in medical school or beyond is charged with having to be compassionate toward you, so you must learn to do it yourself. Whether you are trying to understand a complex case, interacting with patients who have serious medical problems, experiencing an attending's disapproval of you, or struggling to accurately interpret a medical chart, having compassion for yourself will help prevent negativity from affecting your attitude. When you frequently comfort yourself physically, emotionally, and spiritually, you are much better equipped to sustain physical, emotional, and spiritual discomfort in various situations and less likely to adopt behaviors initiated by your false self.

There are a number of techniques you can use to show yourself compassion. One technique is to touch yourself physically. Throughout medical history, touch, or the laying on of hands, has been used as a tool for nonverbal communication with patients. A solid handshake, a pat on the shoulder, a stroke of the forehead, or any other physical connection symbolizes a partnership and expresses compassion and intention for healing. A touch says, *You are not alone. You are under my care. No matter what the outcome of your travails may be, I am here with you and care about you. Put yourself at ease so you can do the work of healing as I help you using the tools of medicine.* Such compassion and intention for healing can also be given to yourself. Imagine that you are not ill but a well-meaning, conscientious medical student who has not yet developed healthy perspective or sufficient skills to grapple in alien environments with patients, doctors, and medical personnel. In the midst of stressful situations or even during daily routines, you can show compassion to yourself through touch. For example, as you move from one patient to the next, wash your hands slowly so that you make contact with yourself, using one hand to stroke, clean, and gently grab the other. Or when talking with a patient or walking down the hall, gently brush one arm with the opposite hand and say to yourself, *I am here for myself.* Or while donning scrubs, imagine that you are dressing in pajamas or an outfit you associate with comfort and your true self. Or take a moment to feel the sensations of nonlatex gloves on your hands or of paper shoe-covers on your feet, and acknowledge how you are protecting yourself. Finally, every time you press the wall button to activate your hospital's double doors, appropriate this sensation to bolster your feeling of groundedness.

Another technique for showing yourself compassion is to replace negative self-talk with healthy objectivity, thus maintaining a realistic perspective on what is expected of you at this stage in your medical training. If you tend to torture yourself with self-criticism, such as saying *I don't know anything* as you are learning, over time you might seriously undermine your self-confidence and ability to assimilate knowledge and perform medical tasks. Or if you berate yourself for inadequacy while under pressure to pull something off for which you lack context, such as performing a procedure you have never before observed, you can make the task even more difficult to accomplish. False messages about your lack of capability strengthen your false self, since the thought of not knowing enough gradually leads to a potentially more damaging conclusion: *I'm worthless.* Instead, remind yourself you are a student at the beginning of your training, and replace criticizing yourself for shortcomings with congratulating yourself on your willingness to learn and determination to succeed. Keeping a realistic perspective on your role as a student with little experience but with potential for increased expertise will help you maintain a connection to your true self. And showing yourself kindness by not torturing yourself mentally and emotionally with scalpel-sharp barbs will make it easier to renounce your false self.

An additional technique for being compassionate toward yourself is to periodically give yourself bits of positive feedback. Give yourself frequent encouragement and congratulatory messages concerning difficult situations and patients, as a ritual to keep yourself consistent and to cleanse yourself of cynicism and morbid fascination—like a self-cleaning oven. For example, intermittently praise yourself for small jobs well done, including learning and connecting with others, and congratulate yourself for successes, however small, especially since such accomplishments are frequently unobserved by others, making self-rewards all the more important. In addition, praise yourself even for effort and courage. For instance, putting yourself out there and asking a good question, such as "How do you gauge when it is safe to move this patient from the ICU to the step-down unit?" is worthy of self-praise. Such feedback acts as positive reinforcement to enhance self-esteem and thus increase your learning skills and boost your productivity.

A further means of showing compassion for yourself is to visualize your future in the medical profession as successful. Just as a patient needs to know his possibilities for future health to muster determination to continue with an onerous treatment, visualizing your future success in the medical profession after overcoming struggles in medical school will give you the resolve to reach this goal and also function subconsciously to help you become the person you are visualizing. For an individual studying primary care, for instance, a helpful visualization might be the following: Imagine you are in your office greeting a relatively new patient you have previously diagnosed with diabetes, hypertension, headaches, and depression. He is a fifty-seven-year-old carpenter who brings with him a picture of his granddaughter as well as a scent of tobacco exuding from his wool tartan coat. You see in his eyes that he trusts you, and he says so at the end of the visit. You ask him to raise the dose of one of his medications, and feel satisfaction when he reports positive results from changes he has made in his life since his first visit, when you suggested that he substitute more nourishing foods for his diet of hot dogs and Budweiser. You shake his hand at the end of the visit and, before the next patient arrives, dictate a brief note to track his progress.

Whatever your chosen specialty might be, create your own visualization of a positive future scenario within it, then use it periodically as a meditation to reduce the stress related to medical school requirements and as an incentive to maintain a positive frame of mind conducive to repudiating aspects of your false self. This is a reliable way to transmute current stress and fears of inadequacy into feelings of hope and satisfaction from anticipated competent and compassionate doctoring.

Finally, an extreme way to help rub away the stray grease-pencil marks of your false self is to deliberately put yourself in a patient's situation to attain a broader perspective on medicine and increase your capacity for empathy with patients. As a case in point, one physician was able to reconnect to the core of his true self after agreeing to be mock-certified, shipped to a state psychiatric hospital for a week, and given antipsychotic medication. Although his ordeal there by no means resembled the frightening scenarios in the film *One Flew Over the Cuckoo's Nest*, nor did Angelina Jolie make an appearance as in her film about psychiatric inpatients, *Girl, Interrupted*, the doctor did have experiences characteristic of such places — such as feeling disoriented, controlled, and fearful. "At first it was fun," he later recalled.

> You're the center of attention and you get a kick from that. But before long you're feeling fear. Sure it's pretend, but still it's a bit creepy and at times genuinely uncomfortable. For me the worst part was that I felt I was being controlled, which did not square with how I 'did' my life — the mandatory jumping through hoops in med school and residency notwithstanding. I discovered that I had no choice as soon as I was shown to my room, later when I was restrained in five points, and during those annoying fifteen-minute checks when I wanted so badly to just get some sleep.

> A surprising transformation occurred within me. As a result of being controlled, I myself felt increasingly out of control. That has brought me down to the level of reality and increased my powers of empathy and observation. And even though those staff members caring for me were more cold and clinical than unpleasant or frightening, still I was distilled down to my core essence — a fragile human being, vulnerable with a capital V.

To get the feeling of being in the situation of a patient on a medical floor, imagine yourself in a bed having to cope with use of a bedpan, the Foley catheter, and surgical team members who fly into your room to interrogate you with such questions as "What were you eating the last time you passed gas?" Such an exercise strips your false self of its veneer and, through increased perspective and empathy, reveals with greater clarity the gold heart of your true self.

A quick way to diagnose and treat emerging aspects of your false self is by asking yourself the following questions:

1 *Are any of my current attitudes or actions negatively affecting my learning process or my relationships with others, especially my patients?* Consider whether any recent occurrence or interaction seemingly derived from your false self. For example, if you asked how to manage unexpected patient erections during physical exams, were you genuinely wondering how to deal with such situations or was it another in a series of attention-seeking, inappropriate questions on loan to you from your histrionic mother? Or have you reinforced your false self by muttering under your breath disparaging but self-bolstering comments about weaker members of your class? Or in your interaction with a patient has your false self encouraged you to act like you know everything in a way that interfered with giving out useful information that might have allayed fears about her impending procedure? The kinds of attitudes you want to focus on are not those that produce simple gallows humor, which at the right time and place can serve as a stress reliever and coping tool, but rather the darker, more debilitating ones that reflect the voice of your false self.

2 *Are my attitudes or actions inconsistent with my true reasons for being in medical school, on this rotation, in this profession? What aspects of them stunt my growth as a medical student, as a person?* After identifying any attitudes or actions derived from your false self, explore their origins, such as the kvetching of your hypercritical father. Reflect on how any new attitudes or be-

haviors may be dovetailing with longstanding unacknowledged emotional wounds that could have opened again in
the medical school environment. Also, since behavior tends
to be reinforced by rewards, ask yourself what you might be
getting out of any such attitudes or types of behavior.

An aid to isolating the voice of your false self can be experiencing it visually through drawing or painting. Equipped
with paper and colored markers, crayons, or pencils, without judgment draw what it might look like. At first you may
only be able to capture abstractions, but as you continue
more concrete images will emerge, the origins of which you
can then further explore through self-reflection. After trac-
ing their sources, you can literally cut out and dispose of the
images to release yourself from their influence. As you toss
them in the wastebasket, or perhaps burn them, say aloud
something like, "I no longer need you. Good-bye!" Making
such a pronouncement empowers your action, giving more
finality to your dismissal of these aspects of your false self.

3 *Where and with whom is my false self most likely to emerge?* The
more attention you pay to your false self, the more you see
which ghosts from the past tend to activate it in a manner
akin to how the powerful Oz created a false specter from behind a thin curtain in *The Wizard of Oz*. Once you have identified scenarios likely to involve your false self, you can practice role-playing them in ways that deflate your false self and
nurture your true self. The more adept you become at anticipating the types of people and situations that might activate
your false self, the more you can prepare for engaging and
then dismissing it. Moreover, the greater your awareness of
its origins and triggers, the better equipped you will be to
observe it yet remain unimpressed by its seductive song and
so refuse to be lured by it.

3 Tuning In to Acting Out

Medical training provides ample opportunity for individuals to lose a healthy sense of reality, become emotionally imbalanced, or undergo disconnection from the true self due to frustration, exhaustion, and challenges entailed in facing medical crises—all of which may lead to acting out. *Acting out* refers to reacting to circumstances in lieu of experiencing the emotions of the moment or simply reflecting on the presenting situation. The stronger the feelings about a situation, the more likely an individual will be to not experience them directly but to react to them. In a medical setting, such reactive behavior occurs most often when there is tension in a relationship with a difficult patient, resident, attending, nurse, or secretary. Usually the person is not aware of acting out until someone tells them they are behaving in an uncharacteristically maladaptive way. Common forms of acting out seen in medical school are avoidance; lying (particularly about physical exam findings); and developing a coldness toward patients.

To understand the dynamics of acting out, it is helpful to look at the physician's relationship to practicing medicine. In medicine we are called to synthesize bits of knowledge into rational decisions and treatments while relating to other individuals. It is important, therefore, to strike a balance between rational and emotional behavior in lieu of acting out. Figure 1 illustrates this

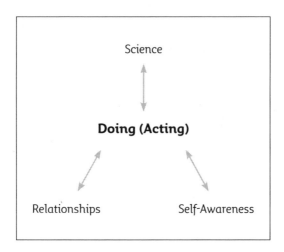

FIGURE 1. Triangle of Medicine: Doing (Acting)

interaction and balance between science, relationships, self-awareness, and doing (acting) — whether you are relating to patients, other physicians, nurses, staff, or the insurance company employee in Arkansas who determines how long your patient can remain on your service.

Medicine is neither entirely science nor strictly social work; rather, it is an artful dance between understanding the scientific basis of disease, dispensing appropriate treatments in keeping with risk-benefit analyses, and relating to patients, family members, colleagues, and relevant specialists. Doctors are in the business of thoughtful, mindful action, but during lapses of self-awareness, such as under personal duress or while acting out, the triangle of medicine illustrated in figure 1 may become unbalanced. When action is guided by insufficient science (for example, medications dispensed without sufficient knowledge or for profit), relationships that cause you to lose good judgment, or unconscious motivations, it is time to look carefully at the triangle and find ways to regain the balance it represents.

An example of how acting out pulls the doing (acting) pole toward the relationships pole would be if you are publicly corrected on rounds by a know-it-all resident after referring to the medicine lisinopril's function as a "diuretic" instead of an "afterload reducer" and in reality feel shame and insecurity. Although you pretend that everything is fine, you behave in ways that are uncharacteristic of you. You might make yourself unavailable, for instance, when the resident needs you to observe a lumbar puncture or assist with an abscess drainage.

Acting out occurs more readily in situations that touch on old wounds originating in the individual's personal history, which accounts for why some people but not others act out in response to a given situation. If, for example, your parents did not give you much freedom to make mistakes as a child, being corrected publicly by a resident might cause you to act out more intensely than someone with more lenient parents.

One extreme example of acting out further shows how such behavior can have its origins in personal history. In group seminars, Sheila always complained, assuming a haughty, dismissive stance toward others, and yet she seemed ill at ease. This behavior escalated until one day, after criticizing the instructor for not providing solid answers to some of the clinical questions posed, she stormed out of the room. Following pressure from the administration, Sheila agreed to see a psychiatrist and subsequently began psychotherapy. During her sessions, she learned to take a mental inventory of issues underlying her bewildering frustration, notably her unhealthy relationship with her mother coupled with the recent death of her stepfather, an important male figure in her life.

Acting out, when unchecked, can cause potentially undesirable or even dangerous behavior, at times destroying relationships with coworkers or compromising the person's education. Even when acting out is used to diffuse tension, and thus does not seem to have negative repercussions, it can ultimately come back to haunt one. A medical school friend who was doing a rotation in general surgery service with his wife, Laura, to minimize the time they were separated after their wedding, related the following story.

The chief resident, acting like a total ass, had a tendency to toss up an X-ray on the viewer and pimp the med students. One time he put up an X-ray and barked to Laura, "What's your diagnosis?" When she answered incorrectly, he yelled, "Wrong!" and punched her on the shoulder.

I was shocked and angry. Later I went to him and said, "If you ever touch her again, I'll fucking kill you."

Then that night from my call room I paged him every half hour just to piss him off. I'm sure he figured out it was me because he changed the call rotation and put me on two nights in a row the following weekend.

While the angry comments were understandable, the pager prank, driven by a desire for revenge, was an instance of acting out. And unsurprisingly, it backfired in the form of more work for my friend.

Medical students can also react to medical situations while outside of medical settings, often acting out through high-risk behaviors. Such acts can be sparked by the need to feel alive and free from exposure to illness and tragedy. The antidote to these types of reactive behaviors is to gain more awareness of their causes and find less risky substitutes that allow emotions to be expressed privately and safely, or stress relieved in harmless ways. For example, Lance signed up for hang-gliding lessons to make himself feel vibrant and capable, in contrast to the helplessness he experienced from witnessing physical debilitation and death on his ER rotation at a level-one trauma center. When his girlfriend made him aware that by hang gliding he was taking risks uncharacteristic of him, he realized that it was an indirect way of coping with his existential angst. Lance caught himself acting out and quit before injuring himself, then eventually found less dangerous hobbies to express his emotions and relieve stress.

To determine if a new and unusual behavior qualifies as acting out, ask yourself the following questions:

1. *What am I doing that is new and different?* Identify any behavior that does not seem to derive from your true self, such as acting passive-aggressively, feeling lonely, seeking attention, or harboring resentment.

2. *Has my new behavior made me feel "good" in the same way an alcoholic might feel relief after taking a few drinks — that is, did the "good" feeling quickly degenerate to regret or cause trouble?* If you are using a certain type of behavior to mask emotions by making you feel temporarily "good," chances are you are acting out.

3. *Why am I behaving differently?* Consider the causes of your new behavior. Is it, for example, because of a decades-long passion for ice-axe solo winter camping and rock climbing, or is it a way to affirm your invincibility and health in the face of all the illness, tragedy, and death you have to confront in medical school? Acting as your own shrink, examine any problem behavior from as many angles as possible, searching for the roots of your actions so you can learn to express the emotions more directly.

4. *What does my triangle of medicine look like right now? Are its elements in balance, and if not, why not?* Consider, for example, the possibility that your decisions — such as postdating prescriptions or favoring one treatment over another because you want the patient (hospital, insurance company) to like you better — are not guided by reason. Or perhaps you are operating with insufficient self-awareness due to a compelling relationship. Or maybe you shrink from dealing directly with a relationship that touches some unresolved issue. Use your insights about personal vulnerabilities to gain increased awareness of any deviations that might cause an imbalance.

If you have determined that some new and unusual behavior qualifies as acting out, or you wish to prevent acting out and thus regain or maintain the balance indicated by the triangle of medicine, the following suggestions may be helpful:

1   Be aware of your vulnerabilities and how these affect your behavior. Becoming aware of your vulnerabilities before even setting foot in any of medicine's emotional playgrounds can help prevent acting out in the first place and assist in coping with acting out later, should it occur.

2   Allow yourself to experience disturbing emotions privately, such as in a bathroom or call room, or among student friends, so that the circumstances causing you pain can ultimately lead to a broader perspective.

3   Use variations of a technique I call "acting in," a coping skill that involves venting your emotions to purge distress. This can be done, for example, by dramatizing (with hand gestures and a script) with a therapist, friend, spouse, or partner. One medical student saw an interesting use of this technique while observing her attending on the orthopedic rotation during an encounter with an unpleasant patient in the outpatient clinic. The physician, a foot and ankle subspecialist, ordinarily had a wonderful way with his patients, able to stroke a foot while doing an examination akin to the best "forehead strokers" — nurses and doctors who populate the critical care wards of hospitals. But this day a patient suddenly stormed out muttering obnoxiously as the doctor began performing pre-op procedures. Once the patient was out of view, the doctor put up his middle finger and directed it toward the chair where the patient had been sitting. Shocked at first, the student soon realized this gesture was a tool the doctor used to relieve emotional stress immediately and thus avoid both repressing his emotions and possibly harming someone. Had he not relieved his dis-

tress, the medical student surmised, he could have brought it with him to the operating room. The student soon learned the value of venting stress immediately and safely to prevent acting out later in some undesirable manner.

Another variation of acting in is to keep a "shadow chart" of your uncensored views as a foil to the regular medical charts you are expected to write. One student, who was criticized for using the phrase "may be tantamount to malpractice" regarding a resident's management of a patient's infection on an internal medicine ward, learned to keep a shadow chart solely for the purpose of relieving the stress that would otherwise build in response to the antiseptic opinions he was expected to write in the real chart.

An additional variation of acting in is the "*Mad* magazine approach." Instead of blurting out something you might live to regret, especially in lecture hall or to your team on the ward, imagine cartoon bubbles above your head containing your comments. Playing out such imaginary scenes in medical settings allows you to defuse your anger or impatience without directly confronting the people who have irritated you.

4 When under stress, reorient yourself by shifting your focus to small, doable tasks or routine chores so that your actions are useful and bolster your feeling of accomplishment but do not cause anxiety or require major decisions. Or reward yourself with time just *being* rather than *doing*, to nurture your true self so you will not feel any necessity to act out. For example, review a textbook chapter, plan your meals for the week, read the travel section of the Sunday paper, do your laundry, go out for sushi or dim sum.

As your awareness of your true self grows, you will become better at assessing behaviors that qualify as acting out in any given situation—in the microbiology lab, in the lecture hall, on the oncology ward, or in the pathology lab. You will also become more capable of understanding situations that touch on old wounds and expressing the feelings that drive such potentially damaging actions.

4

Grappling with Perfectionism & Obsessive-Compulsive Behavior

Although perfectionism and obsessive-compulsive behavior can be useful in academic pursuits, in medical settings they are more likely to inhibit progress and contribute to unhealthy or harmful behavior that can undermine a medical student's career. Liberty is taken here in the definition of both obsessive-compulsive behavior and perfectionism, as most medical students do not manifest the full criteria for pathological perfectionism or obsessive-compulsive disorder (OCD). Nonetheless, medical students can have elements of both perfectionism and OCD, which are likely to be exacerbated by medical school.

Perfectionism, as discussed in *Diagnostic and Statistical Manual of Mental Disorders* (4th ed.), refers to a strong tendency toward orderliness, fear of making errors, and a consuming preoccupation with rules, details, and organization to the detriment of the major objective at hand. Perfectionists are so distracted by the need to control everything that they frequently have unrealistically high standards, handicapping their flexibility, openness, and efficiency. *Obsessive-compulsive behavior*, in contrast, involves repetitive unwanted thoughts, images (obsessions), and actions (compulsions). Compulsions often serve to diminish temporarily the anxiety associated with obsessive thoughts.

Distinguishing between obsessive-compulsive behavior and perfectionism may be difficult because of the clinical definitions used here and the fact that medical students usually lack the full criteria for these pathologies. Within this population, traits of perfectionism appear more prevalent than obsessive and compulsive symptoms. Medical students can fall into obsessive-compulsive patterns without a history of such problems, especially if they have a natural tendency toward perfectionism and are trying to fulfill expectations of precision and competence. Consequently, being on the lookout for either pattern of behavior within yourself will help you maintain access to your true self and improve your concentration, flexibility, and humanness as a medical student. Depending on the kinds of symptoms you experience—such as compulsive hand washing or adopting a rigid approach to managing your patients—you will want to employ specific techniques outlined later in this chapter.

Perfectionism and obsessive-compulsive behavior can cause a variety of problems in medical school. While there are benefits to some repetitious behavior in medical training—evident in such activities as infection-reducing hand washing between patients, repetition of reviewing the gross appearance of lesions (pattern recognition), and daily rounds with patients—students can develop overly repetitious or uncompromising behavior that qualifies as obsessive-compulsive, like fanatically reviewing chart notes, lab values, or patient vital signs. Compulsive behavior can especially cause problems in the operating room (OR). For example, if surgeons feel they have to close every small vein and make sure every last capillary has stopped bleeding before suturing a wound, when standard procedure dictates placement of a tube with negative pressure to draw drainage out, they may prolong the procedure needlessly, therefore abusing the OR schedule or increasing the patient's risk for infection.

Similarly, while accuracy is essential in diagnoses and many other aspects of medical care, perfectionism can prompt overreaction to data. For instance, overreaction to changes in fetal heart rate during preterm labor, without getting supportive data from a sonogram showing that the baby is in trouble, might more easily occur in a perfectionist than in a more mature, mindful medical student.

Perfectionism or obsessive-compulsive behavior among medical students can be caused by a variety of factors. One major cause of obsessive-compulsive behavior in medical school is lack of self-confidence. When medical students are faced with a lot of new information to absorb and techniques to master, obsessive-compulsive behavior can contribute to an ignoring of personal shortcomings. Sally, unsure of her role on her team on the pediatrics rotation, began to champion the cause of preventing latex allergy. Despite the fact that the hospital had already eliminated latex gloves from most departments, Sally kept imagining some poor victim receiving latex gloves and inspected the boxes of them near the sinks outside each patient's room whenever she passed through on rounds. Over time, her obsession with latex gloves led to even more types of compulsive behavior, such as habitual hand washing due to germ phobia. This behavior was a way for Sally to ignore her unease with sick young children who tended to shriek when she examined them.

Actually, lack of self-confidence can become exacerbated in a new environment requiring considerable adjustment, such as a hospital. You may have been adept at filling in bubbles on standardized tests or editing a paper for class, but presenting information to your medical team on rounds may feel so foreign that it can become intimidating and frustrating. Tom, now a hospital physician, remembers how emotionally painful it was as a medical student to do rounds because of his feelings of inadequacy in his new setting. He kept going over in his mind what he had done during the day's rounds. So anxious was he about doing things perfectly that he drove himself crazy. Each time he presented, he felt like running to the bathroom to vomit instead of simply writing, "Mrs. Smith is a fifty-five-year-old insulin-dependent diabetic who was admitted to ICU with a blood sugar of 515, when her husband found her lying on the kitchen floor."

Another, related cause of obsessive-compulsive behavior in medical school is the desire to relieve anxiety, which may be associated with unresolved past situations. It is essential to look out for times when conscientious study becomes an obsessive means of binding anxiety—behavior that reflects not some garden-variety test anxiety, which can help motivate students to prepare for exams, but a potentially more pervasive and harmful existential anxiety. A good example is what happened with Jane, who reviewed her notes ceaselessly and felt compelled to rewrite everything in color-coded block letters using a four-color pen she had saved from her organic chemistry days. But instead of using this method to study more effectively, on an unconscious level she was responding to conditions she had experienced as a child with parents who had been strict about her studies and stingy with praise. Consequently, Jane's obsessive-compulsive approach led her to spend endless extra hours studying, and made her learning a drudgery, with none of the excitement sparked by new knowledge.

A further cause of obsessive-compulsive behavior in medical school is information overload. With so many details assaulting you—abnormal lab results, unclear diagnoses, unexpected patient reactions to treatments—it is easy to succumb to information overload and focus selectively, but doing so can be detrimental to maintaining the broad perspective needed to make optimal assessments and good decisions. Thus, while selectively focusing on one aspect of a patient's problem may alleviate information overload, it can also prevent you from gaining a wider understanding of the patient's medical situation. In one case, Peter, after taking a male patient's pedal pulse but being unable to find one, became obsessed with the man's bony, high-arched, callused feet, wondering if his inability to find a pulse was due to his own lack of skill or the man's poor circulation as demonstrated by the condition of his feet. He was compelled to keep studying the feet until he realized that with thirty-eight patients on the floor he had seventy-six feet to cope with and became overwhelmed. When Peter further considered his peculiar fascination with the man's feet, he realized it resulted from his frustration with the difficulty of assimilating all the information he had been exposed to and from anxiety about being able to perform the rudimentary task of finding a pedal pulse. Additionally, the circumstances reminded Peter of his grandfather, whose diabetic neuropathy was so bad he'd smear a New Mexico chile poultice pad on his wrinkled, veiny feet. The solution to managing selective focus as an escape from information overload is to uncover the hidden meaning behind your fixation. For instance, your fixation may be providing a respite from the anxiety of not yet knowing how to make sense of a case as a whole; shielding you from feelings of inadequacy as you confront so many new medical situations; or triggering the memory of an emotionally unresolved situation in the past.

Excessive focus on detailed information related to medical school can also become problematic in the private lives of medical students. Preoccupation with a million esoteric details from lectures, readings, case conferences, rounds, and chart reviews may lead to loss of perspective and balance. Like an Internet-addicted information junkie, you can exclude most everything other than medicine from your life and thus lose sight of your true self and be unable to recognize when you are acting out. Although medical students sometimes feel guilty if they are not consumed full time with medicine, it is important to realize that such absorption is neither necessary nor healthful. In one particularly vivid case, John became so focused on all the new medical information he was trying to absorb that he couldn't look at a roasted chicken his wife cooked for dinner without analyzing it like something in the gross lab. He picked the bird apart, taking special note of its spinal column and paraspinal musculature. Moreover, their dinner conversation revolved exclusively around medical procedures, such as those involving kidneys or acid-base balance, causing his wife to wonder what had happened to the well-rounded man she had married. Worse still, his obsession with medical information continued in the bedroom, as he envisaged color-coded cross sections of the female pelvis while having sex with his wife. His marriage increasingly suffered as his clinical approach pervaded everything in his life.

An additional cause of obsessive-compulsive behavior is fear of harming others. A student named Bob began compulsively washing, delaying his team from proceeding with surgical procedures as he worried that he might kill his patients by bringing in methicillin-resistant staph. auereus (MRSA). Another student, Vincent, repeatedly made sure the numbers were correct in the little grid box he used to fill in the electrolytes and results of complete blood counts, fearful he might make a clerical mistake that could cause harm. Still another student, Bill, despite already knowing that no major interactions exist between two particular drugs, ran every drug through his Personal Digital Assistant.

Further, fear of harming others physically, or even harming yourself legally, may cause you to be overinclusive about detail in your explanations to patients—for example, turning simple interactions into needless fear-fests by overdescribing all possible risks of a new medication. While major risks need to be outlined, reporting an entire laundry list of potentialities serves to satisfy the provider's need for "completeness" to the detriment of the patient, who, despite the risks, really needs the medication and should therefore be sold on it instead of deterred. Additionally, although you may believe that the longer the list you recite of potential side effects of a medication, the better your protection against malpractice hell, according to some medical legal experts, a long recitation could conceivably hurt your chances in court because it can give the impression that you have neglected to emphasize the *most* and *least likely* problematic events with your patient.

To prevent these and other treatment challenges it is best to nip perfectionism and obsessive-compulsive behavior in the bud now. Another reason for doing so is that given the current medical-legal climate in which physicians must deal with so many reports that include extraneous information to avoid malpractice suits, such behaviors can later seriously hamper the practice of those who have not learned how to control them.

Self-treating perfectionism and obsessive-compulsive behavior is possible using three techniques: speeding up, slowing down, and remembering your humanity. When you are overfocused on one aspect of your work, speed up—that is, get busy with other tasks, such as checking someone's labs, doing a literature search, or seeing what the intern is up to. Even if this feels artificial, it will help you get away from the problematic situation.

Conversely, if compulsive behavior is the problem, slow down, doing whatever is necessary once but thoroughly enough to become satisfied with the results. By slowing down, you can, for example, ensure that the lab values you copied from the computer screen to your cards are correct. This approach—which psychologists Edna B. Foa and R. Reid Wilson, PhD, call the "slow motion technique" in their self-help classic, *Stop Obsessing!*—can be useful in any situation where self-doubt and the consequent need for rechecking and repetition starts to have a life of its own: hand washing, listening to heartbeats, feeling the second "pop" as you perform a lumbar puncture.

The slowing down technique can also entail postponement. If you are obsessing about something you could tell yourself, *I can obsess later, because now I have to see a patient, check to see if the films are read, or find out if my resident is ready to round.* You can do this several times a day, if necessary, and even give the obsession a name to maintain awareness of its existence and harmful potential. Jeanne, now an endocrinologist, remembers using this technique during her psychiatric rotation on a dark ward in a city psychiatric hospital. There was a particularly troublesome and needy patient with mild mental retardation who was so loud and physically large that she couldn't get the image of this hulking man out of her mind even while at home at night in her own bed. She was so obsessed with him that she became physically ill in the mornings, suffering from nausea and headaches. As a result, Jeanne started avoiding this patient, who then became even more needy and would, upon seeing her in the public areas of this small, locked ward, call out her name loudly so that other patients gathered to watch the interaction between them. Her avoidance of him became so noticeable over time that during chart rounds she was mocked for it by her attending. Ultimately, she solved this dilemma by designating time for two meetings a day with the patient and deferring any other contact with him, despite his attempts, to the next specified meeting. Finally, the patient felt he was being cared for sufficiently and even asked to skip some meetings. Jeanne's strategy not only helped control the patient but also allowed her to restrict her obsession with the man to the specified times.

A third technique for overcoming perfectionism and obsessive-compulsive behavior is remembering your humanity, which involves stepping back from situations to view them from the broader perspective of the human condition. For example, Phil, one of the more driven medical students in his class, needed others to think that he was near perfect. As a result, he was highly stressed, especially when others were looking at him, such as during his turn to demonstrate some anatomy in the gross lab. Later, however, when Phil was in the position of being the only Spanish-speaking member of his team while working in an internal medicine clinic and thus had to be the one to tell a Spanish-speaking patient that he was HIV positive and his CD4 count was close to the definition of AIDS, Phil suddenly gained a broader perspective. At that point, he saw his perfectionism regarding trivial details as needless competitiveness in the context of the larger issues of humanity, an insight that helped keep this debilitating behavior under control. Remembering your humanity provides an antidote to unrealistic and potentially damaging agonizing over myriad details, which can lead to errors due to loss of an overview. By contrast, when you maintain a compassionate stance toward yourself and humanity, remembering that life is messy, you are less prone to making tunnel vision–induced medical errors, will grow stronger, and will likely have greater success in medical situations.

The following questions will help you evaluate and control perfectionism and obsessive-compulsive behavior:

1 Are you overfocused on one aspect of your work to the exclusion of others? If so, practice "speeding up" — getting busy with other tasks to regain balance. Rather than fight an obsession, label it and practice postponing reflection on it while saying to yourself, *I'm busy now, but I will think about you later.*

2 Do you repeat tasks, such as washing, checking facts, or mentally reiterating information — behavior that takes precious time and adds little or nothing to your acquisition of knowledge or preparedness? If so, use the "slow motion" technique, performing the task only one time, but thoroughly enough so you are satisfied that you have completed it adequately.

3 Are you so rigid so that you lack any flexibility, or experience rigidity that is inappropriate to the situation in which you are involved? For example, while working in the emergency room, do you have difficulty dropping whatever you are doing to help the next patient in immediate need? If so, first assess your behavior in light of your role models to identify personal traits that may be interfering. Then, to prove

to yourself that you can handle multiple tasks simultaneously and adequately, try doing several tasks at once without
completing the first task before beginning the next. Carefully choose tasks for which there is no danger of negative
results from leaving something partially completed, such as
doing pre-rounds on stable patients.

4 Does perfectionism limit your openness to learning the art
and craft of medicine? If so, just becoming more aware of
this problem can help increase your flexibility and expand
your perspective.

5 Are you overly devoted to work, never able to let go? If so, try
refraining from thinking about medicine for one full hour,
instead reading the *New York Times* from page one to the
end, or pursuing another nonmedical activity. And while at
home, take special care to rejuvenate yourself and nurture
your private relationships.

II

Reinventing Yourself

Part II of this guidebook discusses ways to further expand awareness about the emotional, psychological, and spiritual challenges of medical school and offers tools for initiating personal transformations that can help you succeed in medical school and beyond. Chapter 5, "Bonding with Classmates for Support," addresses how to open yourself up to your peers to discover helpful information about yourself and cultivate allies for support. Bonding with your classmates contributes to decreased stress related to competition and more self-assurance about adhering to your true self when the hospital's environment—from its continuous fluorescent light to possibly difficult interpersonal interactions—warps your emotional judgment. Relationships with classmates can also be beneficial in your later career in medicine by providing a wealth of information about developments in your profession. Suggestions for connecting more readily with your peers are provided.

Chapter 6, "Consciously Creating Your Persona," focuses on creating an identity to present in your interactions with others. Advice is given on how such a persona can be used effectively while dealing with attendings, residents, other staff, and patients. Techniques are included to assess the desired traits of your persona and to create it using a form of role-play.

Chapter 7, "Handling the Difficult Personas of Others," details how to recognize various problematic types of patients and medical personnel, including those who can be aggravating or intimidating enough to impair your concentration and good judgment. It further shows how awareness of such types can help you maintain perspective and efficiency in medical settings. Included are techniques for effectively handling difficult personas.

Chapter 8, "Combating Emotional Shutdown," presents the triggers and symptoms of emotional shutdown and the steps that can be taken to avoid it and remain healthy. Included are ways to gain awareness and develop the healing powers of the self through role-playing with the help of dramas and short stories, one of the most constructive tools for prevention or healing of emotional shutdown.

Chapter 9, "Keeping Dry amid a Flood of Ethical Dilemmas," describes ways to build a personal ethical foundation to support you in approaching difficult ethical conundrums, which abound during medical school and later in a career in medicine. Possible scenarios of ethical dilemmas are discussed and potential resolutions suggested. Exercises are included as an aid to practicing decision making in circumstances where there are ethical concerns.

5 | Bonding with Classmates for Support

To succeed in medicine, you must give up being a driven, competitive perfectionist and form healthy partnerships with peers. Having cleared many hurdles to gain admission to medical school, you can now be relaxed and friendly toward your classmates instead of needing to prove your brilliance. Without peer connections, you will be less effective and successful as a medical student and future physician. Just as the kind of artificial intensity that exists in medical school — one exam after another, a dearth of unstructured time, stressful interactions — has the potential to keep you alienated from your true self, so can it also keep you disconnected from your peers. Remaining socially isolated can result in lack of support in stressful times of study and training, insufficient cooperation during medical crises, and, inevitably, intellectual isolation as a clinician. In reality, the goal of the early years of medical education is not to pass "the test" by any means necessary but to develop skills while working with others so you can remain connected to your true self and also gain training for later association with colleagues and patients (see figure 2).

Medical school can be better than any Internet matching program for drawing together people with shared interests, philosophies, and personality styles, providing great potential for bonding with classmates for support. Just as the body's different organs work in concert toward the same aim — survival and

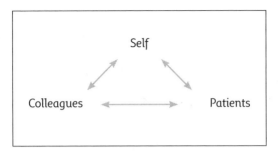

FIGURE 2. Triangle of Medicine: Relationships

growth—so you will need to work together with your peers to gain knowledge, develop skills, and find solutions to medical problems, especially as you become a resident and then a board-certified specialist.

One major benefit of bonding with classmates is support of your true self. When your conduct reflects your true self rather than what you think others expect of you, you are most likely to solidify friendships with classmates who will help you remain true to yourself at times when you may be faltering, such as during a core rotation with irksome residents, when you feel inept because you can't present a case succinctly on rounds, or when a relationship at home is strained the month you are training with a workaholic pediatric oncologist. At times of uncertainty about your views, decisions, or actions, when you are unable to use professors, residents, or attendings as a sounding board, it is your buddies who will remember how you were before the weight of medicine undermined your self-esteem or brought out hints of ugliness in you. Such allies can provide you with a reality check about yourself and authority figures you encounter. For example, one student reported feeling sick while listening to a gastroenterologist, who was lecturing about HIV and AIDS, speak of gay and bisexual men with a judgmental tone suggesting homophobia. After class, the student was able to clarify his feelings with his friends. As a group they realized that, although the gastroenterologist was a prominent figure on clinical rotations and thus unavoidable, they needed to support one another to avoid being negatively influenced by his attitudes.

A second, related benefit of bonding with classmates in medical school is that they can alert you to behavior that may derive from your false self, or provide feedback about ways you might be acting out. Because it is generally easier to see negative qualities in yourself when a respected peer identifies or possesses them, in contrast to a medical elder with whom you do not connect, seeing another medical student act in a maladaptive way increases your chances of recognizing such behavior in yourself and consequently changing your conduct to avoid unfortunate outcomes. In fact, it is often said that qualities that people don't like in others are frequently those that are hidden or repressed in themselves. Undesirable behavior you might adopt includes getting too emotionally attached to patients, not taking care of yourself, and acting self-important to the detriment of relating well with others. For example, Carl was friends with Ian, who seemed to be losing touch with the wider world outside the hospital and often looked sickly, with bloodshot eyes. Worried about Ian, Carl mentioned his observations to him and was startled when Ian responded by saying that Carl seemed distracted and sickly himself, adding that people who live in glass houses shouldn't throw stones. At first Carl was angry and shocked by this response; later, he was able to use the criticism as a springboard to greater self-awareness, sensing that at least part of the reason he had been troubled by Ian's behavior and appearance was due to his own difficulty managing the new stress of clinical medicine.

Another advantage of bonding with classmates in medical school is that doing so can prevent intellectual isolation as a clinician and thus lack of awareness about treatment options. For example, without colleagues to confer with while in private practice, you might not be aware of the experiences of physicians using alternative treatments or of the standard of care in your community. Although it may be hard to appreciate while still in medical school, your social acumen will facilitate critical functions in clinical medicine, such as the ease with which you are able to acquire information, the number of referrals you may get, your ability to access material that could broaden your career, and more invitations to give paid lectures or speak at dinners.

An additional benefit of associating with peers in medical school is that this can help you relate better to patients later and thus treat them more successfully, making it less likely you will face patient dissatisfaction or a malpractice lawsuit. As a case in point, Sandra, an internist who never bonded well with her peers in medical school, later had difficulty connecting with patients as individuals, finding instead that they all seemed to blend together as "them." Moreover, she suffered burnout as a result of her inability to socialize. Fortunately, Sandra made positive changes in her life that fostered better relationships, beginning with a long-overdue vacation to alleviate burnout and later making an effort to have closer contact with her patients during treatment so she could better understand their needs and circumstances.

In another case, Scott, who lacked self-confidence and social skills, became a class nuisance, making his classmates resentful of his need to ask inane questions in lecture hall to bolster his self-confidence. One day, as a lengthy class taught by a long-winded professor was finally ending—with emphasis on the distal nephron's responsibility for fine adjustment of components of urine—Scott posed a complicated, redundant question for reasons unfathomable to his classmates, almost as if he were trying to alienate them. As a result of his lack of consideration for others, he suffered social isolation for the rest of his medical school years and also had trouble relating to his patients during clinical training. The antidote to such neurotic feelings of inadequacy is not to grab attention by inconveniencing others but to confide in peers who are supportive and to forge mutually beneficial alliances.

Yet another advantage of bonding with your classmates in medical school is that you can learn more about a variety of medical specialties from students whose interests differ from yours. Such knowledge can be very useful later, when knowing how a surgeon, dermatologist, or pediatrician thinks might help you make better decisions in your practice. A doctor named Rhonda, for example, found that the friendships she had made in medical school were a great asset in her career. Working as a medical investigator in a pathology department was a perfect career for her, but it was also isolating since she spent hours alone each day examining the tissue and organs of deceased patients. To gain much-needed perspective she began e-mailing her former medical school friends whenever she was stuck on hard questions about an unusual case, and in this way obtained useful information involving different medical specialties that helped her resolve problems. In fact, she received more helpful information than she might have from local colleagues, because she didn't mind sounding uninformed asking her old classmates even basic questions about medical points beyond her areas of expertise, and they felt comfortable answering her without judgment or making her feel ignorant.

For all these reasons, it pays to take relationships with your classmates as seriously as any data you feel might be important for future medical practice—such as the definition of a white count, location of the common bile duct, and problems arising from a patent foramen ovale. Classmates can serve many important functions: making students aware of foibles, acting as a support system, being mentors in addition to the usual authority figures, and later becoming trusted colleagues who can help broaden careers.

Try these suggestions to connect more closely with your classmates:

1 *Lose the competition.* Although among medical students competitiveness is a sometimes-intractable characteristic, it is best relinquished, for it can disrupt healthy bonding with classmates.

2 *Make time for social activity.* A good barometer of your level of pathological "busyness" versus your willingness to develop social acumen is how you answer when medical students ask you to go cross-country skiing with them, or to a movie, or out to dinner. If your answer is frequently, "No, I have to study," consider it a warning sign that you may need to adjust your perspective to include more social activity as a means of realizing long-term goals. Plan a get-together with some of your most compatible classmates and leave the books, lab atlases, and Washington manuals in a drawer at home so you can focus on what makes them — and you — three-dimensional citizens of the world rather than two-dimensional test takers.

3 *Routinely exchange information with a fellow student you trust.* Encourage the free flow of information between you and your classmates by arranging time with one or more trusted peers to review academic or clinical material from a course or rotation. Teaching and learning from fellow students is a good method for testing knowledge, increasing your professional confidence, and enhancing your reputation as a reliable colleague.

6 Consciously Creating Your Persona

Consciously creating a persona enables you to maintain control over the image you project in various medical situations and role-play effectively without feeling like you have sacrificed aspects of your true self. Only in our most secure, intimate relationships (with our lover, spouse, long-time friend, therapist) do we completely expose our true self. In other circumstances, we play roles to a greater or lesser degree. Whereas your innate temperament was shaped by environmental factors during your childhood and adolescence, the image of yourself that you project while among your medical school peers as well as with doctors, or other medical personnel responsible for your training need not correspond exactly with this person you know yourself to be. You were not born a medical student on X rotation; and during your four, eight, or twelve weeks on a certain service it is desirable to adapt to the demands and expectations of the curriculum, medical authority figures, and patients by cultivating the required traits — such as long-suffering patience, necessary to hold a retractor for hours as you assist the vascular surgeon in the second triple-A of the day.

Behaving in a certain way suitable to a given situation, such as blending like a chameleon into the temperament of your team, allows you to perform more effectively with less stress, resulting in more successful outcomes. Just as when making a soup it is advantageous to put certain ingredients in and leave others out so you get a good-tasting broth, you can be selective about the aspects of yourself that you project as you play your role in various situations. In fact, by consciously taking on new roles you are less likely to lose touch with your true self, especially during intense transitions from one rotation to the next, because you protect yourself from emotional pain and anxiety. This leaves you at liberty to have fun in each new position without being so self-conscious and, through self-observation, to learn how your behavior affects others.

To understand better how to develop a persona, it is essential to comprehend the notion of projection—making aspects of yourself outwardly apparent to others. An individual's projected persona reflects internalized concepts of the self and the "other," which are gradually developed over time. Such projection occurs at first unconsciously, when a person begins to develop a sense of self in the context of another person, usually a parent, caretaker, or guardian. When you are very young, the mind's notion of self is indistinguishable from the mind's notion of the other. For example, a hungry, nursing infant apart from the mother feels dissatisfied and unloved, but as time passes and the understanding of self and other becomes better integrated, a child left alone does not experience autonomy as parental abandonment but instead knows that she is still loved, even though the parent is not immediately available.

In adulthood, unless you are conscious of these projected internalized concepts of your persona, and their implications for masking the desires of your true self, unfortunate consequences can result. For example, an anesthesiologist named Lee described how, out of a desire to fit into the group, he imitated his attending's views even when they contradicted his own. In addition, he had a tendency to feign enthusiasm when he had only moderate interest in a subject being presented. On some level, Lee's attending identified with his persona and recognized him as special, while Lee was quick to lose himself in the glow of his attending's admiration. The internalized self reflected in Lee's persona was that of a dutiful, respectful, and love-seeking son, while his internalized other was that of a nurturing, guiding father with only the son's best interests in mind. As a result of this dynamic, Lee chose a surgical residency because his attending said he would be good at it. Lee, forgetting that the persona he projected did not reflect his true desires, took what his attending said at face value and ultimately suffered as a result. Partway through what turned out to be a grueling residency in general surgery, Lee determined that surgery was a poor fit and regretted that he had not remained aware of how the persona he had projected onto his attending was different from his true self-image.

The following techniques can assist you in maintaining awareness of your projected internalized concepts of the self so you avoid their pitfalls as you step uncertainly into the lunar landscape of your rotations and begin consciously creating your persona:

1 Let nothing cloud your view of your feelings and desires. Even when you are excited to discover that you are naturally good at something and important medical authority figures take note, keep an objective perspective and recognize the source of your reaction in the dynamic of obedient child and critical parent. All the while, practice the true-self techniques outlined in Part I and compare your true feelings with those that arise while role-playing.

2 Make two lists, one of aspects of yourself that you like and want to retain, such as conscientiousness and a good sense of humor, and another of qualities that have practical value in medical situations, such as assertiveness in the face of authority, imperviousness to loneliness, and a tendency to workaholism. Commit the first list to memory so you can recall your positive qualities in challenging situations and be able to use them—like small hooks on which to hang

the traits of any persona you create. The qualities on the second list can also be used advantageously, provided that you adopt them to help you achieve excellence and increase your confidence without letting them rob you of your humanity. It is useful on your ER rotation, for instance, to have a kind of amphetamine-driven stamina, but not to the degree that you are an out-of-control maniac.

Now, select the qualities you wish to project consciously as your new persona to help you achieve success in medical situations without losing your inherent qualities you especially like. Be aware that different situations may require you to project different aspects of yourself. For example, a third-year medical student on an internal medicine rotation would want to project different traits than a fourth-year student doing a subinternship or an intern, resident, or attending.

Having envisioned your new persona, role-play aspects of it, by yourself or with a trusted individual, to gauge how others might react to it in different medical school scenarios—a kind of dress rehearsal before performing officially as an actor in the medical school theater. Initially you may want to focus on situations that could potentially evoke fear or uncertainty so you can learn the pitfalls of certain behavior and gain self-confidence in advance of troublesome circumstances. For example, if you are aware that you tend to play the role of overly critical parent when interacting with adolescents, having been primed for this dynamic because of behavior learned from your mother, devise roles that include such scenarios.

It may help to divide your role-playing into two parts, based on the points of view of self and others, as follows:

First, role-play your anticipated reactions to medical situations. To do this, have an acquaintance or partner improvise the role of a patient in a variety of circumstances so you can practice reacting in ways that reflect the persona and qualities you have decided to project, noting how they may vary in different situations. For example, pretend that you are working with a sixteen-year-old girl in the obstetrics clinic who is not taking her prenatal vitamins, continues to have unprotected sex with men other than the father of her child, and still smokes pot and drinks alcohol at parties on weekends. Then determine your reaction to the situation. What attitudes and feelings do you have about treating the young woman? Do you have empathy for her? Do you view her situation more as a medical problem or a social one? What steps would you take to help her, and why?

Second, role-play how you would like to be seen by others in medical situations. Identify the messages you want your persona to convey to the medical staff and patients, and assess the likelihood that these communications will be effectively received based on the qualities you intend to project. Also, change the settings and circumstances to rehearse a wide range of situations involving diverse personality types.

The more you role-play your consciously created persona, the less likely you are to lose awareness of your unconsciously projected persona and the more control you will have over how others react to you and how you progress in medical settings. This way, you will consistently have a hand in your development as you move forward, braiding your increasing medical expertise with growing personal skills.

7

Handling the Difficult Personas of Others

While the intellectual and physical fatigue-related aspects of medical school present anticipated challenges, dealing with difficult people may pose unanticipated difficulties. Hospital staff playing their respective roles (while you are mindfully creating your own persona) may at first appear to be acting with medical wisdom and compassion, but just underneath the surface of this Hallmarkesque scene may lie many unexpected problems, because the actors in this theater may be taking their cues from sources outside the medical setting. In fact, psyche-vexing inhabitants of your clinical world may provide the revelation that dealing with very difficult people is the most taxing component of medical-school life, especially for idealistic and naively empathetic students. Even your seemingly model attending, whose track record of consistently good outcomes makes him the envy of his peers and top choice of patients from miles around, may turn out to be a pathological narcissist whose self-love has gone haywire, making you anxious and fearful.

The usual cast of characters, which includes patients as well as medical staff, is composed of boundary-deficient love seekers, somatizing drama queens (or kings), demanding help-rejecters, petulant parents and adult infants, factitious troublemakers, and abysmal anti-mentors. Following are descriptions of these types and advice about how to deal with them.

THE BOUNDARY-DEFICIENT LOVE SEEKER

The boundary-deficient love seeker crosses boundaries of propriety with such subtlety that he or she causes anxiety and also uncertainty about how to resolve the situation. When someone obviously crosses a boundary of propriety, the inclination is to complain to the individual and, if appropriate, explain what happened to a supervisor, but if the impropriety is subtle, the rectifying course of action is less apparent.

For example, suppose you are treating a man in his thirties for asthma. You greet him in the same way you do all your patients before performing your physical exam. But you notice that when you touch this man's abdomen, he pulls down his hospital pj's, unnecessarily revealing a tuft of pubic hair and a small tattoo. His skin is clammy, as though he were sweaty in anticipation of such an encounter. You wonder if he's just being helpful, although you have a growing sense that he's flirting with you. You experience surprise at viewing this part of his body and also realize that your role as a medical student, unlike that of your "elders," entails an unstated expectation by patients that you will be more like a friend, given your relative lack of knowledge and status in the medical setting. As time passes, whenever you encounter this patient he brings up personal matters, such as inquiries about movies you have seen, some with sexual themes, and where you live. When you act professionally and refuse to divulge information, he makes you feel guilty for snubbing him, showing a facial expression that screams, *I'm hurt by your coldness.* Your emotions become stirred by his verbal and nonverbal pleas for attention, and you wonder if you are being uncaring. Although nothing this patient has done can be proved wrong, his behavior tests the limits of the doctor-patient relationship, making it challenging to find a solution. Yet because he is causing you unnecessary stress and disrupting your learning process, you want to resolve the problem.

Resolving such a situation requires more than simply identifying the man as a sleazy type of individual; it also necessitates examining yourself and learning coping strategies. First, you need to identify any signals you might be unwittingly transmitting or how the man's behavior triggers your feelings of insecurity, causes you emotional stress, or undermines your efficiency on the job. Reflection may lead to a range of conflicting feelings about the circumstances. You may be repulsed by the patient, especially by his apparent unwillingness to play by the rules of hospital culture—that is, by his refusal to be a passive patient. You may find his curiosity about you somehow compelling, or even be physically attracted to the man. Or while he seeks connectedness and feeds off others' insecurity, you may secretly seek approval for excellent work and thus regard his behavior as a flattering substantiation of your ability to relate to patients. Over the course of your soul searching, the patient can actually become a catalyst for self-discovery as you learn about various sides of yourself. In such instances it becomes unclear who is "treating" whom.

Second, to manage this kind of situation you need to employ one of two strategies: using a persona shield or playing dumb. The strategy of using a persona shield means consciously employing a persona to protect you from the emotional manipulation that seems to be occurring. By taking refuge in your persona, it becomes easier to interact with the difficult patient because withholding access to your deeper self enables you to operate without feeling so vulnerable. Whatever touches a nerve can be explored later, after the encounter. While distancing the man by using your persona as mask, insist on sticking with the task at hand, refocusing him whenever necessary. For example, if he drops another non sequitur bomb, you can say, "We could talk about that, but I'm not sure it's going to help your breathing any." The strategy of playing dumb involves acting as though you cannot see through your patient even though you realize something is happening beneath the surface. Using this strategy allows you to ignore inappropriate inquiries and treat them as distractions from your true purpose.

After trying these strategies, recognizing that the patient's persona is very difficult and praising yourself for facing the situation are good ways to give yourself needed comfort.

THE SOMATIZING DRAMA QUEEN (OR KING)

The somatizing drama queen or king is so emotionally needy that regardless of how much care and attention you provide it is never enough. For example, a fifty-three-year-old mother of three came to the hospital with chest pain. The EKG was not compelling, but all her cardiac enzymes had yet to be seen, so a myocardial infarction could not be ruled out. After being admitted, based largely on her presenting complaints coupled with other reported anginal episodes, she demanded unwavering attention, scarcely allowing me to leave the room. At first I felt a certain pleasure at being in the position of rescuer, as there was something endearing about her helplessness, but soon I began to resent her manipulation and see her as a drama queen.

She turned out to be a somatizer, someone who seems to know almost as much about maladies as medical practitioners, speaks medical lingo, and instead of directly expressing depression or anxiety finds substitute relief in medical attention and diagnostic tests. A deficiency of love may be the cause of such a need for medical attention. Encountering a persona like this can pose a conflict for you, pitting your desire for empathic caretaking against a wish to escape from the burden of helplessness imposed on you.

One solution to coping with this type of patient is to learn to tolerate contradictions in people's personas, including your own. If I had not been conflicted about my role and the patient's needs, she would not have troubled me so much, and I could have simply relegated her more easily to the category of "histrionic."

Following is an exercise to help learn such tolerance: List five of your own conflicting qualities, such as "I go to the gym every day, yet I also eat a greasy donut as soon as I get to the hospital." Additionally, list five qualities about yourself that might jar a person caring for you if you were a patient, asking a friend, partner, or spouse to help identify the traits if necessary. Listing contradictory and potentially frustrating qualities in yourself can help you tolerate them in others.

Another solution to coping with this type of patient is to maintain a compassionate stance toward them, and toward yourself for being in a difficult position, while maintaining objectivity in order to limit yourself to appropriate caretaking. In this case, objectively viewing the drama queen with chest pain reveals an ill person with a pathological relationship to herself, whether or not she actually had a heart attack, and thus she is worthy of compassion. You can practice having a compassionate stance toward your difficult patients and toward yourself by imagining such a patient as a family member or envisioning what it would be like to see the world through their eyes. While physical pain may be terrible, emotional pain and its capacity to affect and alienate others can result in even more problems, including loneliness and desperation. Learning to better balance empathy for patients with objectivity, while still maintaining compassion, allows you to perform medical tasks effectively and can help you grow as a medical professional.

Further, even though it is sometimes harder to show compassion for yourself than others, this is important for maintaining balance and perspective in medical school. After all, as a medical student you're often tired, dependent, insecure about knowledge and experience, fearful of evaluation, and accumulating all kinds of debt: financial debt, sleep debt, and free time debt. To begin expressing compassion for yourself, it may help to periodically write short, encouraging messages on a card and make them part of your "pocket library" or tape them to your mini-eye chart.

Alternatively, you can practice self-affirmations regularly to strengthen self-confidence. One medical student used the light-hearted self-affirmation "If only they knew what I know, they'd relax" while looking in the mirror, and as a result his message of compassion became an indelible part of his projected persona, positively affecting his future experiences in medical school.

THE DEMANDING HELP-REJECTER

The demanding help-rejecter demands medical help, but what he really requires for better health is absent from his message to you: a different scenario from that of a noncompliant patient, such as an insulin-avoiding diabetic who nevertheless eats Milky Way bars for breakfast. For example, the demanding help-rejecter might insist you make him feel better but only by using a certain method that he claims works for him, such as the administration of OxyContin, Valium, or some other abusable prescription medication. You know that his history of substance abuse makes use of such medication inadvisable, so you offer a host of alternatives, including more benign pharmacological and non-pharmacological remedies, but all seem unacceptable, making possible treatment not only difficult but frustrating as well.

This type of med-seeking behavior frequently occurs in connection with a habit the patient has no intention of changing. For example, after delineating a litany of techniques you know would help a patient's sleep problems—such as increasing her body temperature so that as she cools she experiences sleepiness or keeping her bedroom dark—you see that her eyes are glazed over and you are being ignored, making you frustrated that your wisdom is being purposefully rejected.

Experiences like this force you to accept that you will not be effective with everybody and will succeed in some cases only at a later time, after the patient has absorbed your words and really wants to be healed. Recognizing that your patient is the one with the problem—or two problems: the presenting issue and a self-destructive hidden agenda—will help you stay balanced so you can provide effective care to the next patient, who may be more receptive to new ideas.

THE PETULANT PARENT AND ADULT INFANT

The petulant parent and adult infant reflect a family dynamic in which parents dominate interactions while their adult children defer to them. Such a situation can cause confusion, making it more difficult to diagnose the individual. For example, a twenty-year-old man came into a psychiatric clinic accompanied by his talkative parents, and it was not evident whether he had a mental illness or only parents who liked to talk. At first it seemed that the personal information they gave about themselves and their son was necessary and desirable, consistent with the more-information-the-better ethos of medical elders, but on closer examination all the information came from the parents' perspective and was thus unreliable. After a while, it turned out the young man was perfectly capable of articulating his own story, although the parents insisted on interrupting. Flanked by them, this young man remained a boy and frequently deferred to their way of looking at the world.

It soon became evident that this family dynamic derived from some unapparent family history or subconscious agenda apart from the young man's presenting characteristics. Even though he had symptoms that could have reflected a potentially disabling psychotic disorder worthy of early intervention, his parents brought along so much additional pathology that it clouded the issues, making diagnosis or treatment recommendations more complicated. Moreover, the parents diminished the chances of a beneficial doctor-patient relationship by simultaneously demanding the best treatment for their son and creating a seemingly impermeable barrier to his diagnosis and healing.

With such a "sick" family, you have made an unwanted purchase—three patients for the price of one—and your solution is to return each item to its proper place on the shelf. In other words, you need to take charge by talking directly to the patient as though he were his own man, and making a diagnosis based on symptoms he reports, using information from the parents only to provide additional context. Chances are the "adult infant" needs you to clarify the family relationships for him and may regard your insight about his family dynamic as a breakthrough opportunity that can lead to both a more accurate diagnosis and an increase in his independence. By not deferring to the dominant parents, you not only refuse to play the "family game" but also dignify your own self in the context of your own not entirely healthy "family dynamic"—the medical system.

THE FACTITIOUS TROUBLEMAKER

One type of patient, the factitious troublemaker, comes to you as a result of having damaged her body or made herself sick. The difference between such patients and others who suffer from self-induced conditions arising from lifestyle choices — pulmonary disease from smoking, liver disease from drinking — is that they have caused self-injury intentionally to get medical attention. The factitious troublemaker may present with any of a number of maladies, such as mysterious skin lesions, patches of missing hair, poorly healed surgical wounds, anatomically impossible loss of motor function or sensation, or full-blown, grand mal–esque "seizures" that have no correlation with EEG squiggles. Extreme examples include patients who surreptitiously inject themselves with potentially lethal amounts of insulin or feces-containing E. coli bacteria, actions taken to fulfill an underlying psychological need.

These patients have a tendency to engender in their caretakers a range of unsettling feelings, from shock to anger to betrayal. You may find also that you develop a kind of perverse Sherlock Holmesian satisfaction from sleuthing and exposing a faker, similar to how one medical student I know gleefully pranced about the dermatology section chanting, "It was factitia!" The "faker" moniker quickly loses validity, however, once you begin to diagnose the patient as truly disturbed.

The principal way to strike a balance in yourself between intellectual sleuthing and caring for such patients is to be compassionate, by looking beyond their physical problems and actions without ignoring them. Also, it helps to forgive yourself for your own feelings of anger or betrayal, which may reflect a passion for conquest over disease or an unwillingness to be shamelessly outsmarted. The most beneficial stance is to maintain a broad perspective and a balance between allowing yourself the excitement of discovery and taking care not to cause the patient unnecessary pain. The key to coping with such a patient, beyond the obvious order for a psychiatric consultation, is to consider it an opportunity to reaffirm that your job is to focus on all forms of illness with equal concentration and lack of moral judgment, in order to help the patient heal.

THE ABYSMAL ANTI-MENTOR

The abysmal anti-mentor is overbearing, arrogant, callous, insulting, and dismissive — the antithesis of behavior you would expect from a mentor. In a medical situation, such a person can be abrupt with patients and lack compassion for them, lecture but never listen, believe he knows everything, and be dismissive toward students and their opinions.

Not only are abysmal anti-mentors destructive to a medical student's learning progress, when they are physicians in private practice they can cause their patients to suffer psychologically and emotionally even as they treat the patients' physical symptoms. Therefore, future doctors need to understand that only in unusual circumstances can a physician get away with being unbearably difficult, such as when they are the only well-published sub-subspecialist of some aspect of medicine within thousands of miles. In situations more subject to real market forces, patients are likely to leave them, and a doctor with no patients does not have much of a practice. For example, one self-respecting woman described letting a doctor's staff know, in the following terms, why she was not making a follow-up appointment: "I hate the doctor, and I'm never coming back. He was rude, arrogant, and he treated me like I was a teenage girl who had her baby out of wedlock." Amazingly, the nurse validated these remarks, answering, "Oh, we get that a lot!"

The key to coping with such a persona is to regard the behavior as a model for how *not* to behave and to encourage yourself, through role-playing, to always provide excellent care for patients while remaining aware of them as human beings with emotions and hopes. You can do this by noting how the anti-mentor relates to patients and observing these patients' reactions, then role-playing in your own mind how you would treat them differently. For example, when you've witnessed such a doctor unapologetically informing a twenty-two-year-old man with adult polycystic kidney disease that his ultrasound suggests the possible need for a transplant—and felt nauseous knowing that in the event such cysts go unnoticed, people often die late in life of other causes—mentally role-play how you would show the patient compassion and advise the least-invasive healing method.

Other forms of mental role-playing can likewise help in dealing with such a person. Imagine, for instance, actually commenting on the troublesome issue with the doctor, your attending, while in the presence of the patient, adopting a Socratic approach employing naïve-sounding queries that subtly reveal his shortcomings, as in the following conversation:

MEDICAL STUDENT: From what I know about this disorder, owing to the anatomic redundancy of a kidney, with so many more nephrons available than are needed for the body to function, isn't it true that adult polycystic kidney patients live long without having a transplant or even dialysis?

ATTENDING: Yes, indeed, that is true.

MEDICAL STUDENT: So, wouldn't it make sense not to treat this too aggressively?

Or imagine asking your attending for advice about announcing such a diagnosis — out of earshot of the patient — in a way that subtly implies disagreement or distaste for his method, such as this:

MEDICAL STUDENT: When you said that to the patient, he looked pained. I wonder how I might break bad news to someone in a gentler way. And I know that "bad" is relative, especially when it comes to these chronic conditions.

Such role-playing will increase your awareness of how you would like to deal with patients while remaining in touch with your true self. It will help mitigate the distress and regret you are likely to experience in other situations with such an attending.

After considering these various types of difficult personas, you can further fine-tune your handling of them by identifying which types cause you the greatest distress and what connection to your personal history might explain their effect on you. Because of their different backgrounds, some medical students interacting with one type, such as an abysmal anti-mentor, may find it a cakewalk requiring negligible emotional energy, while others coping with the same type of persona may find it positively daunting. To develop your own approach more efficiently to such difficult characters, mine your past for situations when you have encountered similar personas. For example, ask yourself if any of your relatives reminds you of the demanding help-rejecter or the petulant parent, or if you have been in a relationship with an adult infant.

Once you make the link between a persona type that causes you distress and a person from your past who exemplifies it, hypothesize why the particular behavior pattern of the persona type is so problematic for you. Ask yourself, for example, how your personality, past experiences, or worldview makes interactions with this persona type difficult. Then focus on changing your reactions to it through visualization and role-playing. For example, envision reacting differently to such an encounter in the hospital. Or imagine the person is someone with whom you have a closer connection, such as a friend, mentor, relative, or partner—who would elicit a different response from you in similar circumstances. Then ask yourself *why* you would react differently to a person closer to you, and adopt coping skills that reflect your new understanding. In this way, you can learn to maneuver a variety of difficult persona types.

Another exercise to prepare for dealing with troubling personas is to create and wear masks that symbolize them. To make such a mask, cut large face-sized ovals out of paper, including holes for eyes, and tape a tongue depressor vertically at the bottom, for a handle. Next draw faces on the masks and write across the forehead of each one the persona type it represents. Then ask a close friend to role-play with you so you can attempt to emulate the thought process of each difficult persona; if you can, in this way, comprehend how they perceive situations according to their psychological and emotional characteristics, you will come closer to devising effective ways to interact with them.

In discovering more about the ways people use their personas in various situations and how challenging certain types of personas can be, you will gain confidence in your ability not only to survive these interactions but also to learn from them. You will also acquire insight into your own vulnerabilities and into the kind of persona you would like to project to medical staff and patients now and in the future.

8 | Combating Emotional Shutdown

The various stresses encountered in medical school may lead to emotional shutdown, a condition that can manifest in different ways, like a hydra with heads of cynicism, despair, loneliness, right-brain atrophy, boredom, and relationship anemia. In medical settings, the resulting shutdown can show up as an inability to empathize with patients or view medicine as beneficial to society. Always, its core is characterized by alienation from the true self. This chapter first looks at the characteristics and consequences of emotional shutdown, as well as its possible triggers, then explores how projecting the self into literary roles, especially through dramas and short stories, can serve as a tool for prevention of or recovery from this malady.

Emotional shutdown, caused by extremely stressful situations, can result in cynicism. When people are in sky-seems-to-be-falling circumstances, their stress hormones surge; their pulse, blood pressure, and respiration increase; their pupils dilate; and their mouths go dry. This classic "fight or flight" response of the sympathetic nervous system can lead to emotional shutdown as a defense mechanism, permitting one to deal with the crisis at hand. Having to confront extremely stressful situations repeatedly over a period of time can result in more prolonged emotional shutdown, in the form of cynicism. Looking at possible scenarios in your own career thus far, if you have examined many babies who are at risk of withdrawing from the heroin their mothers injected throughout their pregnancies, you may begin to view life cynically and question whether good doctoring really brings joy and gratitude, to lose enthusiasm for the remarkable medical advances that might save such lives, or to stop dreaming about the healing you might effect for others in the future. Eventually, you may lose sight of the things that make people human—survival instincts, adaptation to adversity, irrepressible hope for a better tomorrow—and with it the ability to empathize with individuals.

Moreover, the existential angst caused by continually dealing with hopeless people in hopeless situations can bring your potential for optimism down another notch—to despair. You might get your patients "tuned up" so they can breathe better after treatment for their chronic obstructive pulmonary disease, reduce their blood sugar below the scary range, or provide a hospital-based respite from their untenable home situation; but, sadly and frustratingly, you may find that upon discharge they return to the same unhealthy situations: abusive spouses, high-fat diets, chain smoking, sedentary lifestyles, or unprotected sex. Now, the novelty of the situation having worn off, all you can do is remember the effort you put into their cases, arranging for social work or home health care, discharge planning, or getting state approval for Medicaid coverage. Under such conditions, especially if the patients return to your care again on the same rotation, it's hard to remain upbeat about their prognosis or feel like your medical work has value.

Another facet of emotional shutdown is a bitter loneliness. Loneliness occurs when you are cut off from others whose company you enjoy and who give you comfort, most frequently at times of relative inactivity such as evenings or weekends on call, when one blank moment follows another like solitary grains in an hourglass. At such times, with an encroaching insecurity about the merits of your work, you may wish you were at home with your spouse or out on the street. Beneath this longing, as well, you may experience a more fundamental, existential aloneness outside the medical microcosm, a state in which you are not just alone with your own thoughts and feelings but completely lacking the means for validation, self-expression, and interaction with others. You may try to solve this problem by connecting with your patients, but due to their illness or eventual death, you find yourself still totally alone. Forced to take on the biggest issues in life — your sense of self-worth, the meaning of your life and work, humanity's suffering and death — you skulk around the halls, burdened with lack of perspective and alienation from others and yourself.

Another manifestation of, or even trigger for, emotional shutdown is right-brain atrophy or overemphasis on left-brain activity in your work, sometimes due to data overload from graphs, charts, statistics, algorithms, and so on. This can cause tunnel vision, making you lose sight of human issues related to right-brain activity and consequently distance yourself from humanity, experienced as coldness to people or loss of perspective. In addition, instead of entertaining many possibilities, you may see everything in terms of oversimplified dualism — right or wrong, good or bad. You may also feel internal imbalance or emptiness and crave color and aliveness. As the right hemisphere of your brain begins to atrophy from lack of exercise, you may escape to the freedom of fantasy or daydream, but these are mere simple sugars compared with the proteins your hungry self requires for sustenance.

Yet another aspect of emotional shutdown is boredom. Even in the most stressful circumstances it is possible to feel ennui, for instance while collecting lab values, repeating the same questions with each patient, or inspecting the same region of the body as pertinent to your current rotation. As you face another below-the-knee amputation, your zest for medicine may be diminished and you may ask yourself ruefully, *Is this what I'll be doing for the rest of my life?* At such a point, inspiration has taken the last elevator of the evening to the subbasement, leaving you stranded.

Finally, both a sign and a consequence of emotional shutdown is relationship anemia, the crumbling of formerly solid intimate relationships. Such disconnection from loved ones, frequently a spouse, is an unwelcome sign of alienation from your true self. It requires much self-reflection or help from a mental health professional to gain sufficient awareness of the real nature of such a situation, or else you may be fooled into believing that the problems stem exclusively from your loved one and not from your emotional shutdown.

Among the most effective tools for recovering from the insidious yet treatable condition of emotional shutdown is literature, especially dramas and short stories. A growing body of medical humanities literature can address the symptoms and needs associated with emotional shutdown by providing insights into your role in medical school, the hospital, the clinic, or your relationships. Plays and stories may seem an unlikely source of relief from the profoundly discouraging features of this condition, until you realize that most of what happens in medicine mirrors the structure of literary works and can be seen as a dramatization or narrative of the interaction of characters through time — including, of course, interactions between medical personnel or between doctors and patients.

Further, the relationships between doctors and patients are also based on a sequence of actions through time — from diagnosis to treatment to either recovery or death. Even though real-life stories, unlike many well-crafted works of literature, can be frustrating, perplexing, and unsatisfying instead of illuminating, viewing your work in the medical field as metaphorically drama or fiction can help you gain perspective on events and the role your persona plays in them. For example, the constant change you deal with — the shifting of rotations, or a patient's unexpected self-discharge against medical advice — is similar to a tale with surprising twists or one that lacks a familiar denoue-ment. Beginning an ER rotation is like entering in the middle of patients' stories, since it is often only after emergency treatment that you discover a patient's history.

Role-playing difficult personas to learn how to interact with them in medical situations is like trying to understand the mo-tivations for the actions of fictional characters. To better under-stand ways to use drama and stories for gaining insights into your role in medical situations, it may be helpful to learn how other medical students have done this. The following three plot descriptions and anecdotes show how medical students com-prehended medical school difficulties and used them to combat their own emotional shutdown. The first story, Raymond Carv-er's "A Small Good Thing," centers on a young boy who is hit by a car on his way home from school and is brought to the hospi-tal, where he remains unconscious and eventually dies. The story describes the parents' pain, but it is the doctor's discomfort and desire to give false reassurance to the parents as a result of alien-ation from his true self that evokes the deepest angst. In one part of the story, the tanned doctor waltzes into the examining room and tells the parents of the comatose young boy that he is out of danger. Even when, earlier in the story, the doctor seems more human—hugging the aggrieved mother in a gesture showing that he is sorry for her loss—he escorts the parents out of the hospital prematurely, before the mother is emotionally ready to leave.

Another poignant aspect of the story is that the parents have forgotten to pick up a made-to-order birthday cake for their now-comatose son, and the baker is angry about their negligence; un-aware of the tragic accident that has made them forget the cake, he menacingly bombards the family with anonymous phone calls, delivering the message "Have you forgotten about Scotty?" At the end of the story, after the son's death, the mother, having become aware of the source and meaning of the calls, is given a commiserative midnight snack of fresh rolls by the baker, who, although referring to himself also unknowingly gives an apologia for the emotionally shut-down doctor as he admits, "I don't know how to act anymore." While the doctor remains emotionally deficient, the baker is able to respond empathetically.

One medical student remembers how this story helped her combat emotional shutdown. Partway through her third-year rotations, she had begun feeling numb toward the harsh reality of people with illnesses all around her. This student focused her reading of the story on the desperation of people — including doctors — to gain comfort for themselves at the expense of adhering to truth. She remarked, "The poor parents of the comatose kid bank on every word the doctor says, and tragically it turns out what he says is unreliable. As a result of this, I studied my own words more closely, and I looked at my tendency to appease other people, which I knew on some level could lead to my undoing. It's exhausting to have to convince folks that everything is going to be fine when you know it won't be." This student also noted that she now is more attuned not just to the words doctors say to their patients but also to the messages they communicate through body language and gesture, explaining, "Family members are so desperate for the slightest crumb of hope that they try to glean meaning from even the most obscure glance or facial grimace of the doctor."

She wanted to dissociate herself from the emotionally shut-down doctor in the story and instead identify with the more humanistic baker, saying, "I became, over time, more like the baker. I knew I needed to practice medicine with the heart of the baker, not the doctor." If this student had not become more aware of her behavior, she would likely have continued to experience alienation and emotional shutdown.

Another psychologically useful work of fiction for medical students is Thom Jones's "I Want to Live!" This story is about a woman who is diagnosed with cancer, the bad news having been announced by her doctor in an unempathic way. The woman's inner thoughts reveal her fears and pain, as well as her insights on the doctor's alienated self. "The whole problem with him was that he didn't seem real," she reflects. "He wasn't a flesh-and-blood kinda guy. Where was the empathy?" As in "A Small Good Thing," ironically it is someone other than the doctor who does the better job of doctoring and who can empathize with the patient (in this case the patient's son-in-law).

For one medical student, "I Want to Live!" functioned as a salve for his emotional distress and loss of perspective. On his clinical rotations, the student, surrounded by very ill people—particularly people he deemed not old enough to have to deal with cancer—experienced "an emptiness," as he called it, and saw all circumstances as tinged with an aura of meaninglessness. Further, no matter what he was doing, nothing seemed as important as the endless universal battle of healthy-versus-diseased tissue. After reading the story, the student was able to enlist the deterioration and death during his clinical rotation as a focal point for alleviating his emptiness—a reason to celebrate seemingly insignificant sensations and interactions. He remarked, "The writer brings me back from living in a world of black and white to life's vibrant full spectrum."

The student also explained how identification with the fictional patient helped him become more aware of his patients as human beings with inner turmoil, noting, "Her struggle with cancer taught me to read between the lines. I could more easily look beneath the explicit patient responses to questions and just know there is always more under a person's façade." By maintaining awareness of the complexity of his patients' thoughts and feelings, he found a way to regain perspective and balance, commenting: "I was better able to maintain my humor—and stay alive myself during my patients' illness. When I felt that empty feeling creep back into my gut, I would reach for the story and become, once again, not the doctor in it but the life-loving patient, so that I might adapt her intuitive, transcendental understanding of life."

A third story that has offered insight to medical students suffering from emotional shutdown is Ethan Canin's "The Carnival Dog, the Buyer of Diamonds." The story is written from the perspective of a physician who looks back five years to when he came close to quitting medical school, even though he was well into his clinical rotations, because of his relationship with an unusually competitive and stubborn father. By wrestling with both his father's issues and his rationale for wanting to give up on medicine, he gains clarity about his path in life.

A student who benefited from this story suffered from boredom and performance pressure, in response to a mother who pushed her academically. First she identified with the protagonist's difficult relationship with his father, explaining: "My mother was, if not a slave driver exactly, like an activities director on anabolic steroids. She was always in search of the missing two points on the 98 percent I had scored on a math test, and, as a result, to this day I feel uneasy around tests and being judged. Now fast-forward to year three of med school. If you reverse the sex of the quitting med student and his drill sergeant father in Canin's story, that's me and my mother in a nutshell." The story permitted the student to envision different possibilities for her future in medicine. She noted: "I was moving toward family practice and refused to put up with my family's pressure not to become 'only some general practitioner.' Just because my mother had some issue with being the best or making the most money, did not mean that I had to continue, by proxy, to live out her fantasies, I felt. The story gave me a kind of freedom through a glimpse of circumstances that reflected my own wrestling with my mother. I also wondered if on some level in the story, as well as in my own life, the protagonist had a need for rebellion." Ultimately the story made her focus more intently on what she wanted in her life and whether she was accomplishing her goals.

By identifying with certain characters and resonating with evocative themes, you can use such stories to gain perspective and better comprehend your own motivations and goals. To do this most effectively, write comments in the book margins and actively place yourself in the plot, deciding which characters you resonate with and why. Be willing to participate emotionally so you empathize with characters and reverse any emotional shutdown you are experiencing. Also relate the drama or story to your medical training by asking such questions as *What about this story (drama) makes me feel affirmed in my undertaking of medicine?* and *What inspires me to be an excellent doctor?*

Following are additional plays and stories you can use to prevent or treat any emotional shutdown you are experiencing:

» Raymond Carver, "Errand," in *Where I'm Calling From* (New York: Random House, 1988). A story, based on historical fact, about the physician and writer Anton Chekhov. It chronicles the experience of a young man who works in room service at a hotel and is called to run an "errand" for Olga, Chekhov's wife, shortly after Chekhov dies in their hotel room. The young man provides the service and, although nervous about his mission to the mortician, thinks to himself, *I am nearly a grown-up now and shouldn't be frightened or repelled by any of this.* The story demonstrates the difficulties of facing death.

» Andre Dubus, "The Fat Girl," in *Selected Stories of Andre Dubus* (New York: Vintage Books, 1989). A story about a kindhearted, closet-candy-eating, obese young woman that affords an inside view of emotional shutdown. The further the woman strays from her true, even if obese, self, the less connected she feels to those around her, especially her husband. The story provides a window into an overweight person's psychology and, by extension, into the mind of any patient suffering from a chronically unhealthy condition, revealing the contradictions and competing desires inherent in such struggles. This knowledge makes medical students appreciate the fact that patients who may seem one-dimensional because they are identified by their diagnoses are actually complex human beings with likely many unheard heart-wrenching stories, and with whom the students can empathize to avoid emotional shutdown.

» Charlotte Perkins Gilman, "The Yellow Wallpaper," in *Herland, The Yellow Wallpaper, and Selected Writings* (New York: Penguin Putnam, 1999). A story about a woman who descends into madness despite—or perhaps because of—the "help" she receives from her physician husband, who is in a position of authority and does not listen to her. She astutely observes: "John is a physician, and perhaps . . . that is one reason why I do not get well faster." The tale offers ironic commentary on reversal of the physician's role as healer.

» Stellar Kim, "Findings and Impressions," in Stephen King and Heidi Pitlor, editors, *The Best American Short Stories 2007* (New York: Houghton Mifflin, 2007). An endearing story about the bond that develops between a widowed radiologist, as clinical and unemotional as the images he scans, and a thirty-two-year-old patient newly diagnosed with breast cancer. The narrative, loosely structured to resemble a radiology report, traces the physician's reexposure to the cruelty of grief and his transition into wholehearted living and doctoring.

» John L'Heureux, "Departures," in Tobias Wolff, editor, *The Vintage Book of Contemporary American Short Stories* (New York: Random House, 1994). A story about a seminarian in training to be a priest who changes from being unable to tolerate the chaos of people in society to being "removed from them—inhuman." The emotional distance he places between himself and others has a deleterious effect on his relationship with his mother, who dies of Parkinson's disease. The story provides insight not only into emotional shutdown but also into its effects on personality and relationships.

> Bernard Malamud, "The Silver Crown," in *The Stories of Bernard Malamud* (New York: Farrar, Straus, Giroux, 1983). A story that depicts a high school biology teacher's attempt to help his dying father, whose diagnosis is an enigma, by seeking a faith healer. The teacher eventually surmises that the rabbi he entrusted to heal his father from afar might be a snake-oil salesman. The anger and frustration he experiences, he determines, is "what happens when a man—even for a minute—surrenders his true beliefs." This story provides a valuable perspective on the desperate things people do when faced with illness.

>> Shimao Toshio, "With Maya," in Van C. Gessel and Tomone Matsumoto, editors, *The Showa Anthology* (Tokyo: Kodansha International, 1985). A simple story set in Japan about the father of a developmentally delayed girl, who functions for his daughter as a kind of physician. It is written from the perspective of the father as he sits in waiting rooms at a medical clinic. Due to Maya's communication problems, the father is forced to painstakingly and repeatedly ask her questions about how she is feeling, an experience similar to those of medical students interacting with patients who have difficulty communicating. It is clear that, tragically, the father is saddled with these difficulties full time for the foreseeable future. The story prompts medical students to appreciate their less intensive and time-consuming care of such patients, in comparison to interacting with a needy or disturbed family member. It also instills compassion for caretakers dealing with individuals who have developmental problems or communication disabilities.

>> Thornton Wilder, *The Angel That Troubled the Waters* (New York: Coward-McCann, 1928). A short play illustrating how a phy-

sician learns that the anguish of his personal pain becomes his greatest asset in the care of his patients and their families. Sitting around a pool, sick and ailing individuals await the arrival of an angel with curative powers. An able-bodied but emotionally tormented physician summons the angel and is rebuffed by an "invalid" who dreams daily of his own miraculous healing. The angel explains to the physician that the best healers are the wounded and thus he must return to his everyday life and appreciate how his abilities to restore health in others spring from dark places within himself. The drama provides perspective on empathizing with patients as a means of combating emotional shutdown.

9 | Keeping Dry amid a Flood of Ethical Dilemmas

Beyond the gates of medicine lies a veritable hornet's nest of situations that require thoughtful attention to ethics. The life-or-death circumstances so common in medicine—do you or don't you take someone off of life support, continue recommending a feeding tube, increase the morphine—present difficult ethical dilemmas for every person treating patients. Extraordinary circumstances, commonplace in medicine, call for medical students, as members of treatment teams, to have an ethical mooring well before they become primary decision makers. Further, various specialties and sub-sub-specialties—elective cosmetic plastic surgery, for example—by their very nature have the potential to evoke some of life's major questions, such as "What is beauty?" By confronting such questions in medical school, you can gain a more secure foothold along the slippery slope of ethics that you will have to navigate as a physician. Mindful observation of ethical dilemmas all around you, even if your direct participation is limited, provides ample opportunities to fine-tune your own ethical views on a variety of issues.

BUILDING A PERSONAL ETHICAL FOUNDATION

Facing ethical dilemmas in medical school also demands focusing on aspects of yourself that form the basis for your personal ethical foundation. Having the will to do what you think is ethical requires a certain level of awareness of your true self. The inability to recognize such ethical dilemmas may indicate that you lack these requisites and need to reinforce your connection to your true self so you can better develop your personal ethical foundation.

Among the factors that affect how you build your personal ethical foundation are personality and background. Additionally, your background can determine your capacity for perspective—for example, your ability to perceive a broader range of solutions to ethical dilemmas, such as seeing gray areas between the extremes of black and white. And whereas some medical students are more inclined to act impulsively, eager not to prolong an ethical dilemma, others tend to philosophize and seek inner, or even spiritual, guidance. The ethical code by which you were raised, as well as that of your religious affiliation and peers, if you have such, can profoundly influence your current perspective on ethics.

Developing Open-mindedness

In building your ethical foundation for medical decision-making, you should include such necessary components as developing open-mindedness to a spectrum of possible solutions to ethical dilemmas, cultivating an understanding of the ethics appropriate in medical situations, and establishing your own views on specific ethical issues. Developing open-mindedness is important because a doctor's refusal to consider others' ideas and to weigh various options in a specific case can result in needless conflict or even tragedy. No matter what your political or religious beliefs, if you face serious ethical dilemmas with your mind already made up about solutions, you will not be equipped to make the best decisions or optimally serve patients who depend on you for their health and perhaps their lives. No matter how you may ultimately view the ethical landscape before you—whether you would or wouldn't facilitate the withdrawal of Terry Schiavo's feeding tube, for example — each situation requires that you selflessly reflect on the patient's best interest. This, in turn, requires delving into yourself to discover or affirm your personal values.

The following story illustrates how a doctor's lack of open-mindedness can have ethical ramifications by limiting the range of possible options for a patient's care. A pediatrician, born and raised in India, had brought into her practice in the United States many useful ideas derived from her own culture, causing one of her patients considerable distress. As the mother explained,

> She [the doctor] thought that Americans ate too much starch and that babies who started off with vegetables, rather than the usual rice and cereals, would later prefer vegetables and fruits to starches. For my kids this really happened — it was good advice. The trouble came when she insisted that my next son not be circumcised. In the state where I lived, the pediatricians, not the OBs [obstetricians], performed circumcisions, but she refused to do them. She told me repeatedly, "It's unnecessary," and refused to refer me to a pediatrician who would perform the procedure for my son. She even made me feel really bad about wanting it done. In the end, I went elsewhere to have the circumcision done, and I'm glad of it, especially now that circumcision has been found to reduce HIV transmission by 50 percent. Although I liked our original pediatrician a lot, her preaching and close-mindedness made it difficult for me to tell her what I wanted for my child.

In this case, the ethical dilemma was less about circumcision than about the manner in which the doctor commandeered the decision-making process. Disregarding the desires of the mother, in this case, showed an inability to offer her patients a range of choices.

Observing Others and Reading Guidelines

To cultivate an understanding of the ethics appropriate in medical situations, it helps to observe the conduct of other medical personnel in ethical dilemmas, as well as research ethical guidelines of medical associations or specific medical institutions or hospitals. Observing the conduct of other personnel in the medical field can provide an incentive for changing your own personal perspective on ethics and give you a standard for future decision making in specific situations. When doing this, it is important to keep in mind that their decisions may be based on a wide range of resources, depending on the particular person's age, background, and personality type. Other role models can be people outside medical settings, such as parents, friends, and personal heroes. Also, read the standards of hospital ethics boards and the American Medical Association's guidelines for ethical behavior in various situations. While all these resources are important for understanding others' decisions, you will have a greater sense of self-confidence, independence, and integrity if you use them as a springboard for developing your own ethical standards for medical decision making when dealing with patients and others, inspiring you to respond from both your mind and your heart.

Consulting Philosophy

Another good way to establish a context for ethical viewpoints is to study the writings of philosophers who have focused on the subject. One such writer is Aristotle, who noted that in ethical considerations people should strive toward *the good*, a term he used in his *Nichomachean Ethics*. Instead of superimposing your own notions of virtue onto your patients' predicaments, like applying the same label to various blood collection tubes, according to Aristotle a physician "studies the health of man, or rather of some particular man; for it is individuals that he has to cure" (Wheelwright, 166). Aristotle also advised that in feelings and actions a physician should not practice excesses or deficiencies, but rather moderation, striking a "mean." A person in a position of authority, such as a physician, can feel "fear, confidence, desire, anger, pity, and in general pleasure and pain . . . but to feel them at the right times, with reference to the right objects, toward the right people, with the right motive, and in the right manner, is to strike the mean" (Wheelwright, 190–91).

Understanding Science

More contemporary ethics literature, such as Michael Gazzaniga's The Ethical Brain, discusses how an understanding of science can increase your objective reasoning during ethical decision making. Contemporary legal discussions involving right-to-die issues, as in cases associated with the brain-damaged forty-one-year-old Terry Shiavo, can help you gain a deeper understanding and greater legal context for prospective medical scenarios, like a lawyer who studies legal precedents.

Borrowing from Martial Arts Masters

Another way to gain greater perspective for wrestling with ethical dilemmas is to borrow principles from martial arts masters. Consistent with Aristotle's relativism, Shaolin Kung Fu master David Carradine explained that each situation must be considered without prejudice, that it is fallacy to think everything can be "divided into two categories — one good, one evil," and that "strict ethics is pure prejudice if the ethics judge every action in advance" (Carradine, 95). Applied to medicine, this means that medical students and other medical personnel should consider each situation individually and remain open to various possible actions. As in kung fu, where the goal is to encourage the mind and body to work in unison, with neither overpowering the other, in medicine the minds of medical school students and physicians should work in unity with those of patients to avoid conflict. Further, as in Japanese Bushido — a system of samurai ethical principles, one is impelled to follow "a code unuttered and unwritten . . . a law written on the fleshy tablets of the heart" (Nitobe, 35) — "samurai" of the critical care unit should practice meaningful self-control to follow the three essential components of this ethical system: wisdom, benevolence, and courage. And to be at once a reasoned voice of stability while offering a humane hand of comfort, it is essential that medical students and physicians perform "right action" uncomplicated by passion.

REFINING YOUR VIEWS

Once you have a general idea of your personal ethics, you can begin to refine your views on specific issues that will be helpful in most ethically problematic medical circumstances. There are three ways to do this: by thinking broadly, by considering dilemmas through the knowing heart, and by distinguishing between the good and the injurious.

Thinking Broadly

"Thinking broadly" means considering all the subtle details of an ethical dilemma. Thinking narrowly, on the other hand, as if looking at a dilemma through a catheter, offers only minimal, starkly contrasting choices; while thinking broadly provides a spectrum of options. Thus, like a medication that hits many areas beyond the target receptor, a broad approach provides the best opportunity to take an ethical *and* effective stance.

For example, a pulmonologist treating a patient (in the intensive care unit) in his late seventies with metastatic lung cancer was aware that the man had much earlier signed a legal document prohibiting resuscitation and intubation. Despite this, the pulmonologist, upon watching the patient gasp for breath while suffering from bilateral pneumonia, gave him a harrowing choice: "Mr. Smith, do you want the breathing tube or do you want to die?" The patient chose what most would when faced with such extremes — the breathing tube. Once the patient's respirations had calmed and his blood gases had temporarily improved, a medical student on the scene questioned the apparent discrepancy: the doctor, only able to see the man's bilateral pneumonia narrowly in terms of temporary improvement and thus missing the broader picture of his patient's inevitable decline, had contradicted the patient's own wishes stated clearly at a time when he was not in acute respiratory distress. From this limited vantage point, saving the man was a success of some sort, but from a broader viewpoint the doctor's actions constituted an abuse of privilege. Had the pulmonologist assessed the situation within a larger context and obeyed the wishes of his patient, he would have allowed for the patient's continued dignity and prevented additional suffering. A broad perspective invites ethical reflection—you see the forest *and* the trees, the organs *and* the rest of the body, the individual *and* the scenes of his life movie.

Considering Dilemmas through the Knowing Heart

Another way to refine your ethical foundation is by considering the knowing-heart aspect of your true self. This is the screen through which you filter irrelevancies, emotional detractions, and inappropriate influences of others' views on your decision making. To make ethical decisions in medical situations that reflect your true self, you need to entertain the views of others but in the final analysis allow your heart to guide you. You can access the heart's knowledge for guidance through a form of meditation that increases intuitive insights. In times and places of serenity and comfort, such as in a park or on your couch, preferably with the sun shining on you, breathe deeply a few times to quiet your mind, then practice retrieving your heart's knowledge about some medical dilemma by reflecting on your patient as a person, with a life story. Next, add to this story the medical knowledge you are accruing, including the risks and benefits of various potential treatments and the resulting prognoses. Finally, lose yourself and become the patient, with his or her particular needs and desires. After meditating on all these factors, you will be prepared to act ethically and compassionately, like the samurai, even if it results in an "extreme" outcome.

Distinguishing between the Good and the Injurious

A third way to refine your ethical foundation is by gaining greater proficiency in distinguishing between the good and the injurious. This is accomplished by weighing whether action or inaction is helpful for a patient and in what ways. Considering the many permutations of things deemed "good" or "injurious" will often assist you in arriving at a benevolent course of action. The advantages of carefully weighing the good and the injurious are illustrated in the following hypothetical vignette. A twenty-eight-year-old with a seemingly unremarkable history wants rhinoplasty, or a nose job. You meet him with the plastic surgeon you are working with on a fourth-year elective rotation. When you are face-to-face with the pre-op patient, you think to yourself that his nose doesn't look bad, maybe a little bulbous but by no means disfigured. The patient, however, wants his surgery, anticipating the kind of relief that you might expect from the removal of intractably large hemorrhoids. You feel that his not-unattractive nose is unlikely to provide such grief as to warrant having it surgically altered unless there is more to the situation than meets the eye.

Despite your personal doubts, the patient is prepped for surgery, and the nose is transformed. When the patient returns for post-op follow-up, there is tremendous tension in the room. Furious, he expresses deep regret at having had his face altered. Disavowing all responsibility for having elected to undergo this procedure, he vehemently blames the surgeon. The surgeon, however, regarding the nose as superior to the one before and not such a departure from the shape of his patient's original nose that anyone would perceive it as stuck on, à la Mr. Potato Head, feels he has done a nice job and the patient's reaction is unwarranted. In fact, below the surface the man suffers from pathologically impaired self-esteem, a condition not detected during minimal screenings for psychiatric problems prior to the procedure. As an adolescent he had frequently expressed self-hatred while looking in the mirror, telling himself how ugly he was and squeezing microscopic pre-pimples near or on his nose after his weekend shift as a busboy in a greasy restaurant. As an adult, he had generally acted much kinder to himself, except during times of stress when the frayed edges of his tenuous self-esteem would unravel and he would stare in the mirror thinking that his nose was unacceptable and he was worthless.

In this case, the patient's potential surgery could have been better assessed if more questions had been asked in advance to distinguish the good from the injurious. For example, it likely would have helped to query the patient further about how his nose became unacceptable in the first place and why transforming it was so important, perhaps discussing the idea of aesthetic relativity. This case also underscores another dilemma for a doctor—the possibility of reinforcing societal prejudices about beauty at the risk of a patient's physical and emotional health.

IDENTIFYING CHALLENGES

Once you have developed and refined your personal ethical foundation, it is important to identify the most common challenges in medical settings that play tug-of-war with aspects of it due to conflicting priorities. These may include giving patients freedom versus taking control; following personal beliefs versus acting for the good of the patient; and being guided by business and profit and not by altruism.

Giving Patients Freedom versus Taking Control

The first of these challenges, giving patients freedom versus taking control, might occur, for example, when presenting a patient with treatment options according to the informed consent norm, while at the same time specifying which option would be most advisable, considering your role as a provider guided by clinic expertise. Staying true to ethical principles may force you to accept that a patient's choices might not overlap with your suggestions. An example of this is if you become blinded by your own guidepost of total eradication of disease at any cost, feeling a sense of defeat when a patient chooses less brutal palliative care for his cancer, even when the odds of total remission are effectively negligible. Ultimately, good ethics dictate that the patient, the person with the disease, make a well-informed decision about healthcare options much as a judge might render a decision after considering all the evidence and professional testimony presented.

Personal Beliefs versus Acting for the Patient's Good

The second of these challenges, following personal beliefs versus acting for the good of the patient, can easily morph into an ethical quagmire. In general, if your strongly held personal views, including those outside of medicine, contradict what would best serve the patient, good ethical practice requires you to set these views aside. One example might be in the case of a person with alcohol-related liver failure awaiting transplant. You may feel strongly that this individual, despite recent sobriety, has ruined his own liver and thus does not "deserve" a liver transplant as much as an "innocent" victim of a primary liver disease does—a view at odds with what otherwise would be optimal care for the patient. Another example might be that of a deaf individual considering treatment options, while someone you are emotionally connected to in the deaf community is resistant to the use of cochlear implants — say, a close family member who is an advocate for deaf people and feels, as you do, that deafness is not a "disease" requiring a "cure." Your inability to set this view aside could unfairly restrict your patient's choices for improving his own life. In such cases, it is imperative to remember that your voice of authority—as medical student or physician—indeed has power, even if it is only the power of suggestion.

Business and Profit versus Altruism

The third of these challenges, being guided by business and profit and not by altruism, can taint relationships between doctors and patients and subvert ethical practice. For example, in medical situations many subtle motivations exist for using particular procedures, imaging devices, or drugs, any of which can amplify the call for unnecessary diagnoses or treatments. For example, a dentist may "find" areas of concern on teeth and then advise fillings based primarily on her need for cash rather than on the condition of her patients' teeth. Such a questionable ethical situation can occur in any specialty where the procedures are neither risky nor onerous and the indications for them are obvious only to professionals and not patients. When facing such challenges, it is important to remember that ethical practice requires that the primary—if not the only—motivation for employment of any treatment, such as a profitable but unproven radiotherapy device for prostate cancer, remains the eradication of the disease and healing of the patient, not the profit of the physician. Therefore, to maintain an ethical stance, you must not forget that the ultimate goal of the practice of medicine, in contrast to all other trades, is to put itself out of business.

Recognizing the Role of Fear

Today, fear is sometimes used as an incentive to get patients to agree to certain procedures or to taking certain medications. A case in point is a hospital ad I saw recently on a bus, with a confusing photograph and the question "Is this a good freckle or a bad freckle?" Such shameless use of fear prompts the public to search for pathologies and come to the hospital to be tested. To maintain perspective on these types of advertising ploys, it is important to take the context of the ads into account and to be generally aware of how medicine involves a whole spectrum of motivation, ranging from altruism to the capitalist drive for profit.

USING ETHICAL CONUNDRUMS
AS LEARNING EXPERIENCES

Even if you develop an ethical foundation that will prepare you to grapple with these sorts of dilemmas, some circumstances may nevertheless remain problematic, because as a medical student you have limited authority to challenge those in charge. In some cases, you may decide simply to use ethical conundrums as learning experiences, adding substance to your ethical foundation for the future, when you will have greater authority to make decisions consistent with your views.

For example, suppose you are working with a doctor when a patient dies. You are aware that the patient received too much IV fluid for his oxygen count and died from the pulmonary edema he subsequently developed. You also recognize that he was likely to die soon anyway, and therefore the error expedited the inevitable. You accompany the doctor when he meets with the deceased's family, and you do a double take as the doctor tells them something different from what actually happened. At first it appears he withheld information to avoid overly stressing the family. But when they ask if anything had gone wrong during the procedure and the doctor says no, you begin to think he is withholding information to avoid taking responsibility for possible mistakes. In such circumstances it might be best, assuming you wish to complete your rotation, to avoid intervening and instead clarify to yourself how you would have handled the situation. This is not to suggest that you ignore egregious lapses in ethics, but to propose that you carefully weigh factors before deciding to intervene and use situations to refine your own ethical foundation while understanding that medical procedures are imperfect. Or you might resolve to accept the fact that not every situation is as just and balanced as you might like.

KNOWING WHEN TO ACT

In other circumstances, you may feel compelled to contest things you don't like, such as the covering up of a serious error or the omission of important medical knowledge from a report to a patient. For example, imagine you are on your obstetrics rotation and the ob-gyn you are working with is discussing with a patient the fact that her ultrasound shows she is carrying quadruplets, a rare occurrence in the absence of fertility medicine. But he fails to mention the risks to her of carrying all four fetuses to term. You notice the patient nodding and wonder how critically she is assessing the information. Simultaneously, you get a strong feeling the doctor is deliberately withholding information that might lead the woman, in the interest of minimizing risks to herself, to terminate one or more of the fetuses through selective reduction — saying, by his silence, that he is unwilling to perform such a procedure.

Because the purposeful withholding of this information could jeopardize the woman's health, you feel an ethical boundary has been crossed and you might decide to act. If you are inspired to provide the patient with information that will help her make a more informed decision, you might tell her directly that there are other facts she may want to consider. In general, providing patients with options, no matter how grim their situation, gives them a chance to rethink their prerogatives and provides them comfort, even if the hourglass is down to its last few grains. Alternatively, you could question the attending physician's omission of ideas to hear his rationale and philosophy. Or you could share the dilemma with a supervisor you trust and let that person decide on the appropriate action.

SERVING THE GREATER GOOD

A further consideration in dealing with ethical dilemmas is the importance of serving the greater good, which means acting in harmony not only with your own ethics but also with the patient's view of the world. For example, imagine you are alone in the burn unit with a woman in her early forties who, married with two school-aged children and covered with burns, even on her face, whispers to you, "Let me die." There is a living will that demands no extreme measures be taken to keep the patient alive; there is also a durable power of attorney, held by the patient's family members, who, contrary to the patient's wishes, continue fighting to keep her alive. In such a scenario, applying ethical attitudes for the greater good means taking the patient's wishes into diligent consideration.

ACCEPTING MEDICINE'S LIMITATIONS

Finally, it is imperative to learn how to reconcile yourself to the limitations of changing certain medical situations, as well as to unwanted medical outcomes. As a medical student, you have tacitly agreed to participate in medicine, like a patient agrees to participate in treatment, without guarantee of a positive outcome. Recognize that your commitment to medicine entails walking through a veritable minefield of circumstances and unanswerable questions. Ideally, you would be able to change things for the better, but realistically, with so many demands on you, you will have less opportunity to shape the frenetic world of medicine than you might at first suppose. Consequently, except for intervening when you perceive an egregious violation of basic human rights or when common sense would prevent you from sleeping, instead of "fixing" what you notice around you, it is more important to focus on developing a personal ethical foundation that you can rely on in the future. To move forward in your medical life, you need to become adept at accepting less-than-optimal outcomes, even if some of their determining factors go against how you might have handled the situations had you been the attending in charge. This requires that you recognize both the limitations of your power and the fact that many patients entering hospitals are looking for a place to die.

The following exercises will help you practice decision making in medical situations involving ethical concerns and help you refine your ethical foundation:

1 Think of an ethical dilemma you encountered recently. What feelings did it evoke within you? What did you say to someone else about this situation? Were anyone else's views at odds with your own — and if so, how did you handle this difference of opinion? Did your thinking change over time as you considered the details of the case, or as you got to know the patient or her family? Do you think reliance on ideology failed to resolve this situation ethically? Would reliance on your heart's knowledge have allowed you to resolve the dilemma more harmoniously? How could this situation add to your personal ethical foundation and thus help you negotiate future scenarios as a physician?

2 Test market your ethical views, expressing them informally to a classmate or friend who knows you reasonably well. Such a reality check can reveal how your views compare with the perspectives of peers or how your ideas have changed as a result of your recent efforts to connect to your true self. Additionally, you might want to talk about your personal system of ethics in group discussion at the weekly didactics on your rotation, or interview patients about some of these issues to get their opinions about ethics in connection with their own circumstances.

Blazing a Path to Your Deeper Self

Now that you have begun creating the person you want to be, learn how to further empower yourself by operating from within the elemental magma of your unconscious mind through understanding dreams, messages underlying synchronicities, and aspects of yourself linked with enduring patterns, or archetypes, of human behavior. Another important way to take charge of your development in medical school and shape your future is to reflect on your experiences thus far, consciously selecting those that will be helpful for your future as a physician, editing out unhelpful ones, and reenvisioning others to script your own "movie" of your past and future.

Part III of this guidebook focuses

on techniques to increase control over your positive qualities and help you become a successful and compassionate physician. Chapter 10, "Dream Interpretation for First-Time Scalpel Wielders," teaches you how to use dreams to increase the capacities of your true self. By understanding the principal features of dreams and learning how to decode their puzzling imagery, you will better understand yourself and your medical school path. Techniques are provided for interpreting your dreams.

Chapter 11, "Synchronicities, Archetypes, and the Self as Springboards to Spiritual Knowledge," invites you to look at the "chance" happenings and patterns in your life to gain a better understanding of human existence and attain a spiritual perspective. The powerful role of physician warrants a deep comprehension of the context of medicine within life in general. Included are exercises for identifying synchronicities and archetypes in your life and working with them for greater self-awareness and control of your future.

Finally, chapter 12, "Medical School as iMovie: Splicing an Edited Version of Your Self-Story into Residency and Beyond," shows ways to integrate what you have learned during medical school into your later roles as resident and physician. Toward the end of medical school, you have the opportunity to become a "moviemaker," splicing together your most growth-promoting experiences and in the process eliminating those that detract from your future plans. You are encouraged to determine the kind of plot your career-film will take, impacting your choice of specialty and future success in medicine. Included are suggestions for reviewing your past and adapting it for a new movie of your experiences that will help manifest your professional dreams.

10 Dream Interpretation for First-Time Scalpel Wielders

The useful and fascinating insights of dreams can augment your medical education by helping you release tension, understand underlying conflicts and desires, and increase the capacities of your true self. And since dreaming is correlated with intense study, you as a medical student can be expected to dream more than individuals outside academia — that is, if you can get enough sleep.

Scientists have proposed many reasons for why we dream. Sigmund Freud, over one hundred years ago, concluded that dreams display the dreamer's unconscious wishes seeking fulfillment in the theater of the mind. Carl Jung, decades later, felt that the meanings of various dream elements exist on multiple levels, and linked them to universal patterns, or archetypes. More recently, the late Francis Crick, a codiscoverer of the structure of the DNA molecule, suggested that dreams help clear the brain of "obsolete data files," making room for the storage of more current, practical information. According to these scientists, accessing, or "downloading," and interpreting the content of dreams can be an enlightening means of personal discovery that can change an individual's perspective on his life circumstances and on human nature in general.

For medical students, dream interpretation provides an especially appealing method of self-discovery — one that can help them keep focused on their personal paths throughout medical school—since it can be pursued either at home or in the quiet of an call room, using raw material generated in just a few hours of slumberous downtime. Additionally, learning to decipher dreams can lead to profound revelations about conflicts faced in medical school and the nature of one's true self, helping to transform medical school "nightmares" into more pleasant, profession-affirming experiences.

Tapping into raw material walled off in the recesses of the psyche can release not only delights and insights, however, but also unprocessed pain or other unsettling emotions. This potential potency of dream interpretation calls for taking your own emotional temperature before proceeding with this kind of work, which ordinarily occurs in the supportive setting of a psychiatrist's or therapist's office. To determine if you should take a temporary break from this inner work, ask yourself these questions:

1 Have I been feeling alone, detached, isolated, or burdened, as if the weight of the world rested on my shoulders?

2 Have I been dwelling on gloomy, pessimistic thoughts or feelings of melancholy, sadness, or remorse?

3 Am I identifying too closely with the illness, decay, and frenetic distress in the hospital or examination room?

4 Have I been crying or on the verge of tears lately?

5 Have I been losing track of time? Am I losing a sense of myself, or do things around me seem unreal?

6 Am I dangerously short on sleep? Have I been so nervous lately that it's difficult for me to focus or even rest?

7 Have I become unusually irritated, agitated, or angry, causing disruptions in my relationships?

8 Am I sometimes consumed with thoughts of failure, futility, helplessness, hopelessness, or of harming myself?

9 Have I lost my appetite, my interest in daily events, my concentration, energy, or zest for life?

10 Am I using alcohol to quell anxiety, or drinking more than I usually do?

If you answered yes to any of these questions, you may be dealing with depression or a stress disorder warranting consultation with a medical or mental health professional. Plumbing the depths of your unconscious through dream interpretation or any other means requires basic psychological health so that you get the most out of your exploration without harming yourself.

If you are in a state of psychological well-being, dream interpretation should prove more enlightening than unsettling. When interpreting a dream, it is customary to first look at how it unfolds, noting its contents, and then find personal meaning in its special effects. As you engage in such interpretation, you will likely discover some of the intrapsychic effects Freud describes in *Interpretation of Dreams*, especially condensation, displacement, repetition, and wish fulfillment. Although many psychiatrists, including Jung, disagree with Freud's insistence that every dream represents a wish, all believe there are personal messages embedded in dreams — and thus deciphering them can give medical students important insights into their true selves and the reasons for their attitudes and behaviors in medical school.

Condensation is a distillation of two or more beings or ideas from waking life into one image, frequently manifesting as a composite human being. For example, while on your inpatient psychiatry rotation you might dream of someone who combines the qualities of a belligerent patient on the ward and your boyfriend of five years. In your dream, the patient-boyfriend creeps up from behind you and bites your neck. You reach for the wound but feel nothing. Even so, your assailant is surrounded by mental health workers and forced into five-point restraints, whereupon his rage further explodes into scornful disparagements of your authority. Immediately, you decide to discharge the patient. Later, in the chart room, a message comes through the loudspeaker informing you that your patient died. You experience horror, which rapidly gives way to a welcome feeling of liberation. Later, after waking, you focus on the condensation and uncover its meaning: manipulation from your emotionally abusive boyfriend is having an injurious effect on you, preventing you from effectively caring for individuals who require your expertise. You see the dream as an indication that you must liberate yourself from his control so you can be free to express your true self and thus progress along your path in medical school.

Displacement occurs when dream content is oriented toward a feature or action unrelated to the dreamer's waking focus of attention. For example, you may dream about ongoing frustration with antique wallpaper that is peeling and impossible to patch. The more the wallpaper separates from the wall and the more you try to smooth it back on, the more holes are revealed in the surface behind it. Come morning, reflecting on the dream you realize that the image of the peeling wallpaper actually refers to your anxiety about your apparent inability to help heal a patient's wound—an underlying concern that in your dream was displaced onto a home repair job.

Repetition entails a dream element appearing more than once—either in the same dream or in recurring dreams—often in different formats, such as imagery, language, and wordplay. For example, a nearly empty wrinkled bag of Lactated Ringers solution may become omnipresent, seen at first between the cushions of a love seat, then as the canopy of a small umbrella, and later dangling from the rearview mirror of the rehabbed ambulance you drive. The next day you suspect that the bag's recurrence in your dream expresses your depleted resources and a secret wish to relieve your medical school–induced emotional dehydration. It also occurs to you that there might be wordplay at work: your exhaustion from giving to others can be likened to a lactated breast, while the patients, nurses, residents, and attendings may be equated with the bothersome ringers of your beeper.

Wish fulfillment refers to the disclosure of a wish that the dreamer unconsciously wants realized. For example, one medical student preoccupied by the wish to master his desired specialty reported a dream in which he was overseas struggling with the native language and feeling very discouraged about his inability to communicate. Then he pulled a red button from his pocket and pressed it. Feeling something "click" in his head, he suddenly unleashed a torrent of clear communication in the heretofore unfamiliar language. While in this dream the fulfillment is expressed overtly, in others it appears in hidden imagery.

All of these dream elements, if disregarded, can draw you into psychic tumult or leave you with disturbing sensations long after awakening. If, over time, you internalize these dreams while their meaning remains unconscious, they can provoke self-defeating attitudes or actions, as well as unhappiness, as you shuffle disagreeably from patient to patient. On the other hand, you may not be able easily to shake off your uncomfortable sensations from these dreams. In either case, it would be helpful to connect with someone who knows you well, perhaps a professional or an advisor with an understanding of your personal struggles as well as the unique demands and stresses of medical training.

By contrast, practicing dream interpretation can help you access and reinforce your true self, increasing self-awareness. And, the greater your self-awareness, the better your ability to function as a confident medical student, mindful of, rather than ruled by, the hidden agendas of your unconscious. Thus, whereas anxiety produced by a dream may interfere with work, encouraging the emergence of your false self and acknowledging maladaptive patterns of behavior associated with such anxiety can strengthen your true self and keep you on your path. Ultimately, you can learn to dispel the anxiety found in disturbing dreams and use the passion of exhilarating dreams to enhance your waking energy, slipping that excitement into your scrubs pocket like a golden nugget and taking it with you on your rounds.

The following example further illustrates principal features of dreams and how they can be examined and interpreted. Ted, a fourth-year medical student who had just completed an infectious disease elective, had this disturbing dream:

> I'm in a treatment room with the attending, and there's a patient wearing a loose-fitting johnny. Something is horribly wrong with this poor man: he has strawlike gunk in his eye sockets, completely covering his eyeballs. Sweating, he grunts intermittently, his speech basically unintelligible. He is on his feet but leaning forward uncomfortably over a long metal table like the kind on which medical examiners put cadavers. Knowing immediately what to do, I take a sponge and soapy water and scrub his back for him.
>
> The man is at once a patient and my paternal grandfather. I look toward the attending physician, whom I now realize is actually my father-in-law, a doctor in real life, and he nods in approval of what I am doing for this patient. Suddenly discovering that I have not been using gloves, I pull on a pair and quickly return to the work of scrubbing. Now I see that the patient is infected with some kind of parasite. His back is dotted with freckles and small moles. As I scrub vigorously, he says, "That feels good." His words make me feel good, too.
>
> But when I begin washing up, feelings of fear, resentment, and rage come over me, and I ask the doctor if the patient is infectious. "I suppose so," he says. As I pull a couple of brown paper towels from the dispenser, my most horrible fears are realized. There, on my right glove, I spot a little wormlike thing with a bifurcated head standing on its hindquarters and undulating slowly from side to side. The word *fluke* comes to mind, and I instantly see a bunch of flukes attached to my arms. Now

I realize that I will become like this patient, only I will die and my family will suffer. "What a horrible mistake. Why didn't somebody warn me?" I say to myself, feeling a nauseating sensation in my gut.

A close examination of this dream's evocative contents yielded numerous insights into Ted's conflicting anxieties and passions. Ted first identified several special effects, beginning with two examples of condensation. First, the doctor is both a surgeon and Ted's father-in-law, who in real life is a physician but not a surgeon and not hospital based. The second condensation is the combination of the patient and Ted's paternal grandfather, who was obese and, after suffering congestive heart failure and chronic obstructive pulmonary disease, had died prematurely in his late forties. The son, meanwhile, experiences an absence of parenting and of protection from biological danger. In effect, the condensations embody themes relating to family relationships and vulnerability to illness and death.

This dream also exhibits a displacement of anxiety onto the danger of infectious disease. In the dream, the student focuses on scrubbing the patient's back while tragically overlooking the need to protect himself with gloves. The essential action in the dream is a display of altruism gone wrong: the student, or archetypal son, cares for the grandfather, under the guidance of an ineffectual, neglectful attending physician, or father-in-law, who leaves him vulnerable. Ted revealed that he was less concerned about transmission of illness than he was about looking helpful in front of his superiors and further explained that on his clinical rotations he often felt vulnerable himself as he cared for others, especially older men who should be protecting him. The dream thus illuminates Ted's emotional nakedness, a core determinant of his psychic distress.

Further, Ted's dream contains the element of repetition — multiple meanings of the word *fluke*, which is both a chance happening and a flatworm that lives parasitically in the liver, gut, lungs, or blood vessels, attaching itself by way of suckers. Ted illuminated this aspect by admitting that he had struggled with lack of confidence in medical school, including uncertainty about whether he would even be accepted, saying, "I have often wondered if I got in by some 'fluke,' and would say that very word to myself." In free associating about the multiple meanings of fluke, Ted unearthed unconscious meanings embedded in his dream, as if removing the frosting holding together layers of a cake. The associations invited rediscovery of core emotional conflicts that had been stirred up by his new, frenetic life on the ward.

The dream also contained an example of wish fulfillment. The wish in Ted's dream, his desire for an inner sense of goodness and productivity, is fulfilled in the washing of the patient. And the positive feelings this act evokes reflect Ted's exhilaration at helping others as a physician. To him, a true healer involved both being in physical touch with a diseased body and overseeing the patient's course of treatment, both of which are represented in his dream.

In general, interpretation of Ted's dream revealed that he had a pattern of relying too much on protective males in his clinical rotations. As a result, he became more cognizant of his reactions to older men and gradually gained a healthy sense of self-protection, trust in his own judgment, and the ability to take cues from his true self, relying more on himself than his "elders" to determine his physical, emotional, and spiritual safety.

Dreaming of patients, hearing your patients' own dreams, or both, may draw you closer to your true self. For example, a physician had a revealing dream about a patient that increased his ability to empathize with his patients and see his profession in the broader perspective of humanity. His patient, a man in his fifties with dysthymia, low-grade chronic depression, and poor self-esteem, whose same-sex partner dominated when it came to financial and household considerations, revealed a decades-long "dream": to own and operate a specialty restaurant with a set nightly menu and a small but faithful clientele. Despite the availability of adequate financial resources, the man's partner considered this idea "out of the question" and so, given his strong dependency, the patient resolved to abandon this pursuit. One night the doctor dreamed he waited, along with three friends, in the patient's restaurant to be seated. The patient, wearing a three-piece suit and standing at a podium with a small gold bank lamp, indicating his position as maitre d', seemed free from the burdens of his depressive disorder and issues of dysfunctional interpersonal overreliance.

Later, the dream indicated to this doctor his connection to his patient or at least the patient's dilemma and he understood that it offered an opportunity to learn something about himself and strengthen the doctor-patient relationship, but he debated the merits, pitfalls, and appropriateness of sharing his dream's content with his patient. When he ultimately chose to do so, the revelation had a surprisingly positive effect on his patient, who perhaps felt then that his doctor took *his* "dream" (of owning a restaurant) seriously—and that by extension he himself had value. For the doctor, the dream reflected his expectation of good things to come for his patient and the nourishment he himself gained through his work, thus reinforcing how his choice of profession was an expression of his true self.

You can use various methods for interpreting dreams to gain awareness of inner conflicts and strengthen your true self during medical school and beyond. The following guidelines are tailored especially to frenetic medical students, for they encourage deciphering dream images immediately after experiencing them, whether they occur during naps in-house or after hours at home. Wherever your dreaming takes place, instantly focusing on its revelations of your unconscious self helps prevent you from forgetting them in the controlled chaos around you.

1 Place a pen and paper near your bed before going to sleep, whether you are at home or on call in the hospital, resting before being jarred awake by some unwelcome beep or ring.

2 When you wake up from a dream, write down the content as you remember it in a quick, linear way before it fades into the ether.

3 Next, list the important people, objects, and actions in the dream, even if you do not yet recognize their symbolic meanings.

4 Look for condensations, displacements, repetitions, and wish fulfillments in the dream content, enjoying the creations of your unconscious mind as you search for the insights they provide.

5 Then free associate to the dream imagery, noting your first thought or image triggered by elements of the dream, no matter how irrelevant it may seem.

For example, suppose you dream of a plastic speculum behind a glass showcase. This object first reminds you of the day you heard the director of the Metropolitan Museum of Art asking art students to analyze a speculum as an art object visually, purposefully bypassing its functional aspect. This experience in turn triggers memories of your elementary-school art class, rife with rubber cement "boogers," the expression "Haste makes waste," and feelings of being small, messy, and uncomfortable in a smock. Then, with a sudden insight that causes you to fast-forward to the present, you see a connection between the smock and a surgical gown, concluding that the gnawing feelings you have had lately relate to apprehensions about abandoning creativity for medicine's treatment algorithms and compartmentalized manner of thinking and acting.

6 Finally, ask yourself which elements, themes, and result-

ing insights you want to hold on to in your waking life to strengthen your true self—which shells from your psychic sea you wish to keep around your neck as you see your next patient or do your next procedure.

Just as you can keep positive aspects from your dreams to enrich your true self, so you can dispense with dream elements that detract from the vision of who you would like to be. An effective method for doing this is the "nightmare rehearsal technique," a means for "revisioning" a frightening or unpleasant dream, part of which has also occurred in the dreamer's waking life, in order to weaken its power to cause anxiety or other psychic distress. This technique originated with patients "rehearsing" trauma-related dreams in front of a therapist, and gained popularity after British psychiatrist Isaac Marks used it successfully in 1978 to relieve a woman's recurrent nightmare of fourteen years' duration.

To understand how this method works, imagine that two weeks before your obstetrics-gynecology rotation you have the following dream:

> You are in a hospital near the elevators with a group of your fellow medical students. Suddenly a succession of large-bodied people in physical pain—some in casts, some in traction, and others in post-op attire—are wheeled quickly in their hospital beds to the center of this open area, where they ram into one another, making crashing noises. As this happens, an elevator opens and you dash inside; but when you push the black "tongue" along the side of the door to keep it open for your classmates, it cracks apart, reminding you of an unhealthy placenta. The door then closes abruptly, pinching one earpiece of your stethoscope and ripping your white coat pocket, out of which falls a small address book with a disturbing image on the front of a baby with mongoloid facies

emerging from a birth canal along with the faces of the horrified parents. You realize you are personally responsible for this tragedy and experience self-loathing.

Based on the self-loathing you feel while dreaming, you conclude that the birth of this child with Down's syndrome to ill-prepared parents is somehow linked to your poor practice. Two weeks later, part of this dream recurs several times during your obstetrics-gynecology rotation, forcing you to reexperience your impression of yourself as a klutz with a reverse Midas touch—in a position of responsibility but contributing to a disastrous outcome. You are not yet fully aware that your nightmare amplifies a host of personal anxieties you have sublimated in your waking life: concern about your capabilities as a medical student; difficulties with the chaos around you in medical situations; uncertainty regarding the use of medications, as represented by the black "tongue" in the elevator door; and, ultimately, worries about your responsibility for bad medical outcomes.

In working with this dream, you first implement the six steps outlined earlier to determine its meaning. Then, in response to the need to release its powerful hold over you, you use the nightmare-rehearsal technique, revisioning elements of the dream related to personal attributes and subsequently practicing them in waking life. For example, revise the dream in your imagination by going back in time to the patient's prenatal care and seeing yourself as the practitioner who performs the amniocentesis and receives the karyotyping results. At this point you could envision finding that the chromosomes are normal and there is no Down's syndrome, or see yourself discovering the trisomy at chromosome 21 and helping the parents cope by explaining their options. After revising the dream in your imagination, "rehearse" the revised dream sequence before bed. As a result, the medical nightmare will cease, because the new, emotionally nourishing content reflecting your conscious wish fulfillment as a physician has become absorbed into your mind, simultaneously decreasing your anxiety and enabling confidence to spring from your true self. By using the six-step approach plus the nightmare-rehearsal technique, you can "doctor" your true self and your vision of the type of physician and healer you wish to be.

As you record and explore the possible meanings of your dreams, it will become increasingly evident that, contrary to recaps of the medical TV comedy *Scrubs*, dreams are not "pleasure visions" whose purpose is to restore exhausted medical students so they can perform well when their pagers beep them back to conscious awareness. Rather, dreams are useful tools for helping people to understand their underlying conflicts and desires and for activating and nourishing their true selves.

11 | Synchronicities, Archetypes, & the Self as Springboards to Spiritual Knowledge

During your core rotations as a medical student, you may often be forced to confront major issues of suffering and death that prompt you to see such medical circumstances in the larger context of humanity, beyond any medical ward. Continually managing patients with serious medical problems or on the verge of death may eventually cause you to hunger for increased spiritual knowledge. Consequently, it is helpful to explore some ways of attaining a broader, more universal perspective on aspects of your true self and your endeavors as a medical student. Before beginning this inward quest, plant your fingers firmly on your emotional pulse to evaluate the solidity of your emotional framework. Because work of this sort can exacerbate an already tenuous reaction to stress, it necessitates good psychological functioning, and therefore ordinarily happens at the end of one's psychotherapy, once core issues have been expressed and exchanged for an integrated, sanguine perspective.

SCANNING FOR SYNCHRONICITIES

One way to see situations with a broader perspective is by becoming familiar with theories about the occurrence and meaning of specific personal events in relation to the more universal view of humanity. For example, Carl Jung believed that when certain events intersect in a person's life they have special meaning beyond ordinary reality. Such synchronicities, as Jung called them, reveal information about your true self and deepen your connection with the spiritual dimension. Robert H. Hopcke's book *There Are No Accidents: Synchronicity and the Stories of our Lives* offers numerous stories as examples of synchronistic events. The implication is that although not every synchronicity signifies a life-changing moment, some do, and by heeding their signs and discovering their meanings for you as an individual, you will emerge with the broader perspective of a spiritually enhanced physician.

Ironically, the more attuned you are to synchronous events, the more they seem to occur, as when you learn a new word and later encounter it almost everywhere you go. Indeed, in medical school the awareness of synchronicities is really an extension of a faculty for pattern recognition that can help you align with your desires as they intersect with everything the universe presents to you. With this enhanced perception of synchronicities, even small, seemingly insignificant events become potentially meaningful guideposts.

Synchronous events are most obvious when they incorporate a strong emotional component. For example, Cindy, after a year of anguishing over her inability to conceive a child, and experiencing agonizing miscarriages and fertility clinic consultations, first saw a human birth during her obstetrics-gynecology rotation as a third-year medical student, and this synchronicity made her look within herself for its deeper meaning in the context of her life. She recalls her experience in the birthing pavilion:

> I had no idea what would really happen until there was the head and all the incredible excitement. No longer an abstraction to me, here was this beautiful skin surrounding this live creature, with eyes that were looking around. Not yet a mother myself, I realized that only here and now — unless I chose to specialize in OB [obstetrics] — would I be able to experience the first moment of a baby's life from this angle. I wanted to savor the experience, especially at times when my identity as

a medical student did not feel life affirming. When a healthy baby is born and you're a part of that, it makes you consider your own existence and connection to nature. For me this vicarious experience was especially poignant considering what I had longed for in my own life. I felt as though the young mother knew intuitively how I had suffered in recent months with multiple miscarriages. This feeling was enhanced by the fact that the in-house attending on duty that night was the same fertility specialist who only days before had outlined my own options for successful conception of a child. Dealing with the dual role of being both medical student and patient to my supervising attending constituted a minor footnote compared with the enormity of this coincidence in my life.

Both the pain and the exhilaration accompanying her experience of this synchronicity caused Cindy to become more spiritually conscious, as if birthing her own "spiritual baby," functioning as a bridge to the deeper intuitive self and the spiritual realm. By not dismissing this coincidence as meaningless, Cindy was able to transform her resentment about dashed personal hopes into a broader universal perspective that allowed her to consider a possible future in obstetrics.

Finding Meaning in the Ordinary

A career in medicine provides a magnet for synchronistic events since it involves a lifetime of encounters with people. Through whatever trajectory—you're the only neurosurgeon for three hundred miles, or you were randomly chosen from a list of preferred providers on a patient's insurance company Web site—such meetings can result in synchronistic events that may have significant implications for your own current circumstances. For instance, you diagnose a patient with the oddly named Jumping Frenchmen of Maine disorder the day after booking your flight for a Montreal conference and ordering a

CD to learn French; years later you are reminded of this patient in your evaluation of a diagnostic conundrum and home in on the correct diagnosis, using it as inspiration. Through such experiences, you appreciate the hidden interconnections between human actions and world forces, as well as the potential meaningfulness of even the most banal encounter. In so doing, you open up a door for exploration of the spiritual dimension.

LOGGING ON TO AN INTERNET OF ARCHETYPES

Another way to help broaden your perspective enough to create a bridge to the spiritual dimension is through an awareness of archetypes and their meanings. As a medical student, your intimate view of the cycles of life, illness, and death connects you to universal human patterns or archetypes, which, according to Carl Jung, stem from the collective unconscious, a kind of psyche shared by all people throughout history. Like an individual's personal unconscious, the collective unconscious exists beneath the level of everyday awareness; but unlike the personal unconscious, it is available to every human being and the archetypes therein are inherited, not requiring personal experience for their existence within one's psyche. Jung made clear, the mind cannot be "localized" in space but instead connects with the greater psychic universe, providing archetypes and synchronistic phenomena (Campbell, 518). To understand this better, imagine a dispersion of small bits of primitive information swirling around the World Wide Web but with your mind, rather than a computer, as the portal through which you tap into this psychic framework. This "mental Internet" includes all feelings, experiences, and thought processes common to humanity in general. Further, the recurrent, timeless aspects of human behavior and experiences within the collective unconscious manifest concretely as different archetypes.

As a medical student, you can become aware of archetypal roles linking you to the collective unconscious, enabling you to increase your effectiveness in medical situations and practice medicine with greater spiritual awareness. This makes even more sense when you consider how doctoring and the spirit have historically been combined. For example, in his famous oath Hippocrates invoked the physician god Aesculapius, who became so powerful that he successfully brought the dead back to life, signaling the importance of viewing medicine in a larger, spiritual context. Learning to see medical actions more in terms of playing archetypal roles thus helps give you a universal perspective, so that as you defibrillate your patient during a code you realize you are symbolically enacting the Aesculapius myth, bringing healing energy from the spiritual dimension, thereby adding to your capacity for compassion and healing.

Of the numerous different archetypes you might potentially encounter as a medical student in hospital, clinic, and office settings, the following represent the ones that seem often to emerge among medical students and doctors in medical settings: the warrior, the priest, the great mother, the king-father, the magician, the obedient child, the scribe, the person of science, the ambulance driver, the feeder/disturbed chef, the vampire, the know-it-all, and the futurist.

The *warrior archetype* represents the qualities of the quintessential protector and fighter, and a person embodying this archetype often acts according to the kind of automatic response behavior required in rescuing—like the preconscious reaction of the man between the rails of the New York City subway, who, without taking time to think, saved another man by protecting his body with his own. The warrior archetype acts instinctively in the service of preserving life or health, but without regard for consequences.

The *priest archetype* encompasses aspects of a leader, a magician, and a healer. This archetype embodies both decorum and mystery. A human link to the divine, the priest uses ritual and the laying on of hands to effect cosmic insight and spiritual healing. Medicine's various rituals, structured settings, and guidelines provide a good environment for the priest archetype; the medical student, via this archetype, should be able to connect more easily to the spiritual realm of healing.

The *great mother archetype* represents fertility, nurturing, and comfort. This archetype reflects the kind of comfort and healing that springs from nature.

The *king-father archetype* has the qualities of solidity, inner strength, and benevolent love, evoking the kind of deep understanding that only maturity and confidence provide. This archetype also appears in the context of protecting, rule making, and benevolent leadership, emphasizing the notion that the kind of power it imbues in doctors and doctors-in-training requires judicious application.

The *magician archetype* reflects skill in the arts of transformation and transmutation through illusion and alteration of appearances. This archetype may appear in connection with doctors who remove cysts or abscesses, as well as those who use sedatives and anesthesia.

The *obedient child archetype* embodies subservience, craves attention, and struggles with independent thinking. You might have a tendency to strongly identify with this archetype as you seek positive feedback from your teachers, just as you might have for years before the first clinical rotations in medical school. Aligning yourself with this archetype might be useful at first but quickly loses value once you realize you need to consider cases independently and rely primarily on yourself for emotional support.

The *scribe archetype* represents obsession with details and lack of ability to see a broader perspective. Tireless pursuit of "only what's important" for the test or clerkship evaluation not only blinds the scribe from seeing context but also results in lack of enjoyment.

The *person-of-science archetype* is connected to observation and categorization of the world. This archetype takes refuge in organization, lists, and logic, and pursues intellectual mastery and left-brained understanding. The person of science does not relate to the chaos in the world but instead looks for order in everything, including human behavior. This type would be nonplussed by the view of life portrayed, as it is by one contemporary musician, as "a pigsty."

The *ambulance driver archetype* is characterized by the tendency to help in any crisis. Needing to take charge, this type focuses on emergencies, but lacks a long-term view of situations.

The *feeder/disturbed-chef archetype* nurtures — but to a fault. In contrast to the great mother, the feeder tends to relinquish self-care in the process of caring for others, and the radical version of the feeder is the disturbed chef who might err on the side of killing with kindness. In an extreme example, the disturbed chef might continue to give tube feeds to a point where the patient's stomach overflows with the excessive "nutriment" and he begins to aspirate the material into his lungs. The character Jack in the television series *Lost* provides another example of this archetype. His single-mindedness in preserving life can also cause him to overdo commitment and neglect an equally important feature of mindful doctoring: letting go.

The *vampire archetype* thrives in the context of others' failure, discomfort, or disability, all of which boost the vampire's self-esteem and level of functioning. An example of this archetype is a psychiatry resident who bolsters his own low self-esteem through contact with individuals "sicker" than he considers himself to be.

The *know-it-all archetype* repels people and so remains isolated and lonely. Medical students who align with this archetype lack meaningful connections with peers and tend to pursue a career path that requires little interaction with patients and colleagues. Clinics, state institutions, and academic centers often attract this type.

The *futurist archetype* is so focused on the future that she does not enjoy life in the moment. An example of this type is the medical student who is excessively concerned about being the resident or attending down the road and is unable to enjoy learning.

Recognizing archetypes as they appear in various situations and comprehending their potential effect on circumstances can help you gain awareness of the collective unconscious and thus deepen your relationship with the spiritual realm. (For a more general look at archetypes, see Carol Pearson, *The Hero Within: Six Archetypes We Live By*, or Robert Moore and Douglas Gillette, *King, Warrior, Magician, Lover: Rediscovering the Archetypes of the Mature Masculine.*)

One Medical Student, Multiple Archetypes

The following anecdote illustrates how one medical student used knowledge of various archetypes to achieve mystical insights into herself and the world.

Emily, a third-year medical student who was about three-quarters through her inpatient psychiatry rotation at a state psychiatric hospital, became sufficiently confident to lead the morning treatment team meetings as well as the walk rounds immediately thereafter, though still under the guiding eye of her attending physician. Her growing confidence was dashed, however, when her attending criticized her comments to a manic young patient. Emily, who was only a few years older than the talkative, energetic, hypersexual woman, spoke earnestly as she told this woman how "young, attractive, and vulnerable" she was and how her "exposed midriff was just asking for trouble" in the surrounding population of confined, predominantly male patients. After Emily forcefully doled out this heartfelt "advice," the attending insisted on seeing her in the private conference room, where he warned her: "Never, ever tell a manic patient that she is very attractive. It eggs her on and makes things worse. Instead, your task is to assess her mental status and connect with her so that she might accept meds and improve sufficiently for a safe discharge."

This criticism made Emily reflect on her motivation for speaking to the patient as she had. On some level she knew a greater force was at work, but only after uncovering archetypal aspects of her life in medicine could she understand it. At first she noticed that in her interaction with the manic patient she had aligned with the so-called warrior archetype and thus transformed herself into an avid protector of a vulnerable young woman. This warrior archetype has a pragmatic place in medicine, especially in the battle against invading cancer cells, the protection of children from sexual abuse, and the slaying of the dragons of disease and disorder—whether medical, surgical, or psychiatric. Emily's alignment with the warrior archetype could have been helpful or harmful depending on the situation, but blind submission to it could also have prevented her from learning the appropriate way to deal with certain types of psychopathology and thus could have narrowed her medical perspective and made her ineffective.

In an uncanny moment of synchronicity a day later, Emily was aligned with an unusual archetype for her—the priest archetype—thereby balancing her lopsided orientation toward the warrior archetype. Emily aligned with this archetype when a hulking male patient—whom she had had in mind when she had advised her female patient the day before—suddenly handed her a small statue of a woman with the name "Dymphna" etched on the base, saying, "I need you to protect this for me."

Conferring with her attending, Emily learned that (Irish Christian) Saint Dymphna was the patron saint of mental illness. Receiving this statue suddenly made Emily perceive how powerful she was in the eyes of patients, which oriented her more toward the spiritual dimension. Reflecting further on the hidden meaning of the scenario, Emily realized that receiving the statue of Saint Dymphna was a starting point for a new understanding that there were universal elements in her work related to the collective unconscious and that she was playing many roles on her psychiatry rotation, including those related to the archetypes of warrior, priest, magician, healer, mother, and father.

After this insight, Emily was able to see her patients in a new way—according to archetypes relevant to situations—and was better able to balance contrasting tendencies in her work. As a result, she became more effective on the ward and gained the kind of spiritual knowledge essential for enlightened doctoring.

EXPANDING INTO A SPIRITUAL DIMENSION

By scanning your medical school life for archetypes and synchronicities, you can expand your true self into the spiritual dimension and thereby gain strength to use in healing. For example, Jack, a fourth-year medical student who had grown up outside of any formal religious tradition, felt free to explore various spiritual practices and recognized an invitation by a Hopi ward clerk as a synchronicity worthy of his exploration. This woman suggested that Jack purchase a whole cantaloupe to bring with him to a Native American pueblo's annual Corn Dance. Intrigued, Jack bought a round, unblemished melon, placed it beside him on the passenger seat of his car, and made his way to the celebration. While walking around the festival grounds carrying this intriguing sphere, Jack meditated on its many different symbolic meanings, imagining it could be a human brain, a disembodied cadaveric skull, or an enormous ovarian tumor.

Using the cantaloupe as a focal point, by the end of the day Jack had discovered that his connection with the spiritual realm originated in his inner self. Then as he stood in a stranger's house with people he had never met before, at a cultural ritual that was new to him, eyeing a gorgeous spread of food while experiencing a feeling he could only describe as "freeing," Jack became transfixed by the slicing of his cantaloupe offering. Initially sliced in quadrants, he saw these pieces as directions and areas of his life—where he was headed, where he had been, what was outside himself and what was within—while the seeds seemed to represent his potential as a physician and the origins of his spiritual growth. He realized also that the search for self, especially in connection with archetypes, ultimately is a search for spirit.

Viewing your circumstances in medical school from a universal perspective, and thus connecting to the spiritual realm, can lead to psychological and emotional healing, which is especially valuable during times of personal struggle. For example, when you realize how many mundane tasks, such as checking blood pressure for the umpteenth time, accompany day-to-day doctoring, you may feel like the novelty of practicing medicine has devolved into drudgery. Treatment for this condition might include looking at the universal context of your work to regain inspiration and a sense of your work's value. Much as a Buddhist monk might use daily tasks, like cleaning, as a vehicle into the spiritual realm through humility and meditation, your repetitive and mundane jobs during medical training need not disintegrate into Sisyphean rock pushing but could likewise be a means to a higher consciousness.

Another time that you may need spiritual healing through gaining a more universal perspective is when you realize you have a deeper connection to your patients' charts than to your patients. With so much emphasis on documentation, the inanimate three-ring binder of papers and, worse, the virtual chart of the computerized record can easily become perverse replacements for the actual people who desperately need your help and expertise to heal. Because of the medical-legal environment in which U.S. medicine is practiced, often medical students bear the emotional brunt of fear-mongering by their "elders" and thus many expend too much energy making charts look beautiful at the expense of examining patients or educating themselves about diseases. Given these circumstances, it is useful to consider how you may be identifying too closely with such archetypes as the person of science and how identifying with another archetype, such as the king-father, could help change your perspective and make you feel more connected to a universal context.

Yet another circumstance that may require spiritual healing through a broader perspective is when you feel alienation from your work and your true self, or a kind of existential angst about life in general. This state of mind can occur, for example, in the early years of medical school while you are learning about a natural cellular process known as "apoptosis," or programmed cell death, a process we can live neither with nor without: in its absence, cells grow unrestrainedly as with deadly cancers, while with apoptosis we have what might be called a "shelf life." When looked at this way, life becomes a true double-bind, a catch-22. Such a discovery can give an already demoralized, burned-out medical student a sense of hopelessness. Instead of succumbing to nihilism—which might seem the natural course after dealing continually with terminally ill patients—seeing your work in the larger context of the spiritual realm can be life saving. To heal yourself as you work with such patients, align yourself with the energy of the priest archetype; nourish yourself as would the great mother archetype; and expand your perspective, as would the futurist archetype, by taking a long-term view of meaningfulness of your profession in the years to come.

A final example of how seeking a spiritual connection through a universal perspective can be invaluable to a medical student is the following scenario. While on a certain rotation, you feel that you are not getting a handle on some basic idea—such as under what circumstances for a given cancer you would use radiation therapy alone versus surgical intervention, chemotherapy, and then radiation. Your bewilderment leads to low self-esteem and doubts about your aptitude for medicine; yet these difficulties are occurring in the context of your prior aptitude for absorbing concepts of treatment algorithms, such as those for hematology and oncology in your second-year sections. Given these facts, you can see that your current struggle likely has less to do with your intellectual capacities and more to do with the condition of your psyche and its connection to the spiritual dimension.

Consequently, as you contemplate your circumstances, teachers, patients, and attitudes, you may notice connections to relevant archetypes. For example, you may realize that you have identified with the feeder — caring for everyone but yourself, so that now you do not feed yourself intellectually. Your task, then, might be to try to align with the person of science archetype and reclaim your footing as a competent medical student. By becoming aware of how your circumstances reflect specific archetypes, you gain insights into the possible origins of problems, as well as see your situations in a multidimensional context. In instances of lingering low self-esteem or persistent melancholy, distress, or negative thinking, augment or replace the archetypal route to personal healing with real-life connections to individuals who know you well.

By focusing on various archetypes that surface through your medical work, you further deepen your view of the self and expand your spiritual capacity. Seeing interactions as more universal than the details of the moment links you to events stretching back millennia in human history and provides a way to value more fully your role in medicine.

The following exercises will help you identify synchronicities and archetypes in your actions. Use them to deepen your relationship with your true self, your connection with the spiritual dimension, and your ability to see your role as medical student and physician in a broader context.

1 Think of a time recently when an uncanny coincidence occurred. What personal message did it convey? How can you
   use the meaning of this coincidence to better understand
   your inner self and your connection to the spiritual dimension? How can you more vigilantly keep an eye out for future
   synchronicities as they emerge in your medical training?

2 Which archetypes tend to appear when you are working
   with patients (residents, attendings)? How might you align
   yourself with specific archetypes to work in a more effective
   or balanced way? How could invoking certain archetypes in
   your work bring you closer to your spiritual center and empower you as a healer?

3 Think of a recent experience that provided you with an opportunity to develop your connection to the spiritual dimension. Did you take advantage of the situation at the time it
   occurred? If not, can you now use the insights to develop
   your spiritual awareness?

12 | Medical School as iMovie

*Splicing an
Edited Version of
Your Self-Story
into Residency
and Beyond*

Toward the end of medical school, having focused on some of the approaches suggested in this book, you will have accumulated not just information about diagnoses, treatments, and surgical procedures, but considerable knowledge about your true self. If you think of your mind as a type of camera, such self-knowledge consists of many film clips stored in that camera; these clips are the raw footage you can edit to make a montage or intrapsychic DVD, as though you were using a mental iMovie editing tool as you reflect on your experiences. You can then store this DVD to use as a resource for even greater self-knowledge and guidance in the next phase of your life as a physician.

At this early phase in your career, you have a choice: either you take time to edit your iMovie or just let all the fragments of medical school memories remain unedited, a record of the moment-to-moment banality of your life, akin to a convenience-store closed-circuit security video. The better option is to reflect consciously on all your medical school experiences, editing your "film clips" into a useful montage that contains the essence of all the things you have learned about your true self, your goals, and your connection with the spiritual dimension. In this way, your experiences become a learning tool you can refer to later to sustain your self-confidence and personal vision as you embrace the challenges of your upcoming residency and postresidency professional years.

Editing and splicing together this mental movie of your experiences requires reassessing past attitudes and actions, reinforcing positive memories, revising negative ones, and selecting or omitting such memories to create a film that supports your maturing self and your ultimate professional goals, a process that is similar to the one in chapter 6 for consciously creating a persona from chosen aspects of your character. Not only is the end product, the movie, valuable to your developing self and career, but the process of editing can itself be highly educational. Psychologist Dan P. McAdams underscored the educational value of stories when he remarked, "Stories are not merely 'chronicles,' like a secretary's minutes of a meeting, written to report exactly what transpired and at what time. Stories are less about facts and more about meanings" (McAdams, 28).

Thus, you can use the process of editing to gain insight about your past desires and behaviors, assessing your growth from the film clips selected for your movie and also from those you decide to discard. With each such assessment, you essentially refine your understanding of your goals and the personal qualities and learning experiences crucial to achieving them.

Editing the story of your medical school experiences not only provides enlightening information to bolster your future success but simultaneously heals emotional and psychic wounds resulting from all the challenges and stress of medical school. By including particular experiences, you consciously reinforce the positive aspects of your life as a medical student while eliminating the influence of negative experiences; this is why the editing process can help heal emotional and psychic wounds.

For example, instead of retaining an unsettling experience of being unable to count on the resident to do the right thing—after he did not respond quickly or seriously enough to a man with marked bradycardia before the attending physician gave you both a lesson in cardiology and shame, undercutting your already tentative self-confidence—you can now revise this unnerving episode by accepting it as a no-longer-painful, invaluable lesson about conscientiousness in doctoring. By leaving the self-defeating film clips on your mental "shelf," while clicking and dragging the valuable clips into the movie, you save only the knowledge useful for your personal and professional objectives. What may seem at first like revising history is actually a means for cultivating a future in which you can have greater self-awareness and be more psychologically balanced, compassionate, and morally strong. The truth of the past is not ignored but only recontextualized so it can become a more useful tool for you in the future. In doing this, the clips that didn't "make the cut" in your movie are not lost but rather archived for replay and reevaluation if needed, either as reminders of your former self or the paths you decided not to take—invaluable "waste" that could yield critical information about the self at some later date.

For instance, imagine you are back on your inpatient psychiatry rotation where you first experienced an acutely agitated female borderline patient requiring five-point physical restraints as well as a shot of Haldol, Ativan, and Cogentin, a cocktail of chemical restraint. As you and the attending order this treatment, he explains how the scene comes as close to rape as permissible by law. You then feel disgust at the whole scenario. Unless you plan to be a psychiatrist, the film clips of this unpleasant memory may now be relegated to the shelf of video shorts which you've determined to be of negligible relevance to your tightly edited movie, although they may be retrieved at some later time, if necessary, such as when you have to treat a difficult psychiatric patient.

Editing to revise your experiences in such a way that old wounds are healed will assure that the final version of your movie can strengthen your true self and your ability to deal with potentially painful medical situations in the future. Even if you have been fortunate enough to avoid major traumatic situations during your training, small chinks in your armor can undermine self-confidence and drain energy needed for good doctoring. One wound that is painful for many is a memory of having not had the correct information to adequately diagnose or treat a certain patient. In one case, a medical student observed interviewing a patient on a medical floor found himself unwittingly pretending to know some bit of information that was later proved untrue. In his assessment for delirium, the medical student mistakenly took the patient's mention of goat heads to be visual hallucinations of heads of goats instead of little, irregular-shaped thorny burrs, and unwilling to experience embarrassment by admitting his ignorance, came to the wrong conclusion about the patient's mental and physical state. The memory of this scenario remained a painful reminder of his inadequacy, largely because asking questions and not taking things at face value is a core aspect of a good doctor. Looking back, however, the student was able to revise the story and give it a broader context, highlighting what he had learned about the need to ask questions rather than assume knowledge of a subject. Thus all such events from early in your career can become lessons learned, while the negative emotions and energy attached to them can be diminished or eliminated. Without conscious revision of such memories, you might not have a broad, mature perspective of the past with which to face the future.

Once you comprehend the value of editing to create your own movie of the past and become adept at revising the negative film clips, you can also learn how to give your movie a clearer plot and structure so the action progresses logically according to character motivations. By making a movie that includes your best aspects and goals, you will be able to reveal behavior and attitudes that might more easily impact your future decisions, such as your choice of a specialty. Your specialty can be selected with more authority when you have edited your memories of medical school, because such an important decision needs to be based on a thoughtful perspective of your long-term passions and life philosophy rather than on momentary desire. If you employ soul-searching editing techniques in creating your movie, your specialty should be naturally revealed to you and help you retain interest in your future.

When you are ready to decide on a specialty, ignore all the advice you may have received about pursuing an area in which you would not likely be replaced, since, once you create your movie so it supports your goals positively, you will necessarily become irreplaceable in any specialty. In the end, it is best to pick a field about which you are passionate; otherwise, you may double your resentment each time you call the pharmacy, the nurse, or the OR. One art history professor's advice to prospective graduate students was to not bother pursuing an advanced degree or specialty unless "you cannot sleep because you are so taken by a specter seen in a dark corner of a Velásquez painting" or are similarly passionate about some objective that overshadows your daily existence.

Finally, to reinforce your goals, "film" your future by imagining yourself as a character in your movie. By filming the future in this way, as if it were already a reality, you can direct your intention toward personal and professional success, thus helping ensure its manifestation. For example, film yourself practicing your choice of specialty with patients you treat successfully, such as a middle-aged woman who, after a reprieve from a low-grade depression she has suffered from for a long time, is liberated to enjoy herself in ways she had not in years. Or picture yourself ensconced in a comfortable office chair, medical diploma side by side with other certificates of merit on your office wall, as you lean back to take a break from your dictations and replay what you have just stated into your microphone: "Lesion successfully removed. Complications: none." Further, imagine that this patient is just one of hundreds of people whose lives—because of your expertise and clinical acumen—you have dramatically altered for the better. Also imagine, perhaps, that you have just discovered something new in the course of clinical research, leading to a novel tool for the medical treatment of certain autoimmune disorders. You could also film yourself in your chosen specialty, able to manage various complications when they arise and feeling intellectual, emotional, and spiritual satisfaction knowing your work means something not just to you but to fellow humans as well.

While visualizing such scenes, embrace the future self you imagine with confidence that the situation will manifest. Then live your life now as a medical student in concert with what you expect to experience later.

As you create your own movie, consider the following activities as ways to enhance its production:

1 Review your life over the past four years, reflecting on how you have changed. Write down the most vivid scenes for your film clips.

2 Reviewing the film clips, decide which are important for continued strength and growth and thus, even if they caused pain or unease at the time, should be included in your movie, as well as which detract from a positive future and thus should be revised for inclusion or omitted.

3 As you mentally replay the new montage you have created, identify major themes that provide structure to the movie's plot. Determine how these themes may be an expression of your true self or your goals for the future.

4 Decide what kind of theme music your movie should have and how this reflects your true self and your strengths.

5 Determine who and what to list in the credits at the end of your movie, to show the influences on your positive development in medical school or before—inspirational people, books, or events significant to the building of your personal perspective or ethical foundation.

As you practice using the tools described in this book, you give yourself a variety of gifts. At times the gift might be large — such as discovering or learning more about your true self, revealing, possibly for the first time, under a light brighter than any that illuminate operating rooms worldwide, the brilliant gold heart beneath the tarnish of your false self. At other times the gift might be smaller and more subtle, like a new ability to handle difficult colleagues or patients, or sticky ethical dilemmas requiring thoughtfulness and personal restraint. Your exploration of stories illustrating deeply personal accounts of common experiences within the realm of medicine can be a tonic to help soothe your emotional shutdown. Additionally, you may open up paths you had not previously considered — such as exploration of your spiritual dimension and connection to the collective unconscious — for increased perspective and strength. And you may affect your career positively by editing the film clips of who you are today, all the while envisioning yourself as successful in scenes of the future. Finally, you give yourself one of the most significant gifts when you deeply know this truth: I am and will remain a capable, empathic, ethical, spiritual, and mindful medical student . . . as I move into my new life as a mindful physician.

bibliography

Adler, Mortimer. *How To Read a Book*. New York: Simon and
Schuster, 1940.

American Psychiatric Association. *Diagnostic and Statistical
Manual of Mental Disorders*, 4th ed. Washington, D.C.:
American Psychiatric Association, 1994.

Barrett, Deidre. *The Committee of Sleep*. New York: Random
House, 2001.

Bulfinch, Thomas. *Myths of Greece and Rome*. New York: Penguin
Books, 1985.

Campbell, Joseph, ed. *The Portable Jung*. New York: Penguin
Books, 1984.

Canin, Ethan. "The Carnival Dog, The Buyer of Diamonds."
In *Emperor of the Air*. Boston: Houghton Mifflin, 1988.

Carradine, David. *Spirit of Shaolin: A Kung Fu Philosophy*. Boston:
Charles E. Tuttle, 1991.

Carver, Raymond. "Errand." In *Where I'm Calling From*. New York:
Random House, 1988.

———. "A Small, Good Thing." In *Where I'm Calling From*.
New York: Random House, 1988.

Coles, Robert. *The Call of Stories: Teaching and the Moral
Imagination*. Boston: Houghton Mifflin, 1989.

Crick, Francis, and Graeme Mitchison. "The Function of Dream
Sleep." *Nature* 304 (1983): 111–14.

Delaney, Gayle. *All about Dreams: Everything You Need to Know
about Why We Have Them, What They Mean, and How to Put Them
to Work for You*. San Francisco: HarperSanFrancisco, 1998.

Dubus, Andre. "The Fat Girl." In *Selected Stories of Andre Dubus*.
New York: Vintage Books, 1989.

Dyrbye, Liselotte N., Matthew R. Thomas, Jefrey L. Huntington, Karen L. Lawson, Paul J. Novotny, Jeff A. Sloan, and Tait D. Shanafelt. "Personal Life Events and Medical Student Burnout: A Multicenter Study." In *Academic Medicine* 81, no. 4 (April 2006): 374–84.

Foa, Edna, and Reid Wilson. *Stop Obsessing!* New York: Bantam Books, 1991.

Freud, Sigmund. *Interpretation of Dreams.* London: George Allen and Unwin, 1923.

———. *Introductory Lectures on Psychoanalysis.* New York: W. W. Norton and Company, 1966.

Friedman, Martin. *Close Reading: Chuck Close and the Artist Portrait.* New York: Harry N. Abrams, 2005.

Gazzaniga, Michael S. *The Ethical Brain.* New York: Dana Press, 2005.

Gilman, Charlotte Perkins. "The Yellow Wallpaper." In *Herland, The Yellow Wallpaper, and Selected Writings.* New York: Penguin Putnam, 1999.

Hopcke, Robert H. *There Are No Accidents: Synchronicity and the Stories of Our Lives.* New York: Penguin Putnam, 1997.

Jones, Thom. "I Want to Live!" In John Updike and Katrina Kenison, eds. *The Best American Short Stories of the Century.* Boston: Houghton Mifflin, 1999.

Jung, Carl G. *Dreams.* Princeton, N.J.: Princeton University Press, 1974.

———. *Memories, Dreams, Reflections.* New York: Vintage Books, 1963.

Kabat-Zinn, Jon. *Wherever You Go, There You Are: Mindfulness Meditation in Everyday Life.* New York: Hyperion, 1994.

Kim, Stellar. "Findings and Impressions." In Stephen King and Heidi Pitlor, eds., *The Best American Short Stories 2007.* New York: Houghton Mifflin, 2007.

Laing, R. D. *The Divided Self.* New York: Pantheon Books, 1969.

L'Heureux, John. "Departures." In Tobias Wolff, ed. *The Vintage Book of Contemporary American Short Stories*. New York: Random House, 1994.

Malamud, Bernard. "The Silver Crown." In *The Stories of Bernard Malamud*. New York: Farrar, Straus, Giroux, 1983.

Marks, Isaac. "Rehearsal Relief of a Nightmare." *British Journal of Psychiatry* 133 (1978): 461–65.

McAdams, Dan P. *Personal Myths and the Making of the Self*. New York: William Morrow and Company, 1993.

Miller, Alice. *The Drama of the Gifted Child: The Search for the True Self*. New York: Basic Books, 1997.

Moore, Robert, and Douglas Gillette. *King, Warrior, Magician, Lover: Rediscovering the Archetypes of the Mature Masculine*. New York: HarperCollins, 1990.

Moyers, Bill. *Healing and the Mind*. New York: Doubleday, 1993.

Nitobe, Inazo. *Bushido: The Soul of Japan*. Tokyo: Kodansha International, 2002.

Pearson, Carol. *The Hero Within: Six Archetypes We Live By*. New York: Harper and Row, 1986.

Pogue, David. *iMovie 2: The Missing Manual*. Sebastopol, Calif.: The Pogue Press, 2001.

Roberts, Gregory David. *Shantaram*. New York: St. Martin's, 2003.

Schwartz, Barry. *The Paradox of Choice: Why More Is Less*. New York: HarperCollins, 2004.

Siegel, Bernie S. *Love, Medicine and Miracles: Lessons Learned about Self-Healing from a Surgeon's Experience with Exceptional Patients*. New York: Harper and Row, 1986.

Singer, June. *Boundaries of the Soul: The Practice of Jung's Psychology*. New York: Doubleday, 1994.

Toshio, Shimao. "With Maya." In Van C. Gessel and Tomone Matsumoto, eds., *The Showa Anthology*. Tokyo: Kodansha International, 1985.

Van de Wetering, Janwillem. *The Empty Mirror: Experiences in a Japanese Zen Monastery*. New York: St. Martin's Press, 1999.

Wheelwright, Philip. *Aristotle*. New York: The Odyssey Press, 1951.

Wilder, Thornton. *The Angel That Troubled the Waters and Other Plays*. New York: Coward-McCann, 1928.

Winnicott, D. W. *Home Is Where We Start From*. New York: W. W. Norton and Company, 1986.